SIRT FOOD
The Secret Behind Diet, Healthy Weight Loss, Disease Prevention, Reversal & Longevity

The Medicine On Your Plate – Vol 1

By John Hodges & Ted Gif

www.viddapublishing.com

Cover design by John Hodges.

VIDDA Publishing BOOK SHELF:
www.viddapublishing.com/books.html

Have you thought about self-publishing via Amazon Kindle? If so to make the process easier and more productive, I highly recommend this software to help you on your way.

KBookPromotion: http://jvz1.com/c/391033/167361

Your FREE Gift

Thank you for purchasing this book. To show our appreciation we would like to offer you a FREE copy of our eBook: "**A Complete Handbook of NATURE CURES**".

To download, go to **http://viddapublishing_0.gr8.com/**

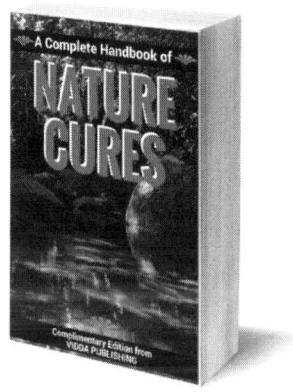

If you're interested in Health, Nutrition, Green and / or Cruelty Free products please visit our Websites and online **VIDDA Health Store:** astore.amazon.co.uk/vi07a-21

www.viddapublishing.com

www.sirtfood.com

www.themedicineonyourplate.com

www.greenupyourlife.org

www.ecologizatuvida.com

Table of Content

Introduction

"Out of clutter, find simplicity. From discord, find harmony. In the middle of difficulty lies opportunity"
Albert Einstein

It is probably fair to say that most of us have never heard of the term Sirtfood and to be fair there is no reason why we should have. This book is not an exhaustive analysis or even partial critique of the biology of Sirtfoods or the proteins they are hypothesised to activate. It is more to impart that eating Sirtfoods is not a fad and that the action of SIRT proteins is the subject of detailed research by agencies which are engaged with seeking solutions to conditions ranging from cancer to Alzheimer's disease. You do not need a biology degree to understand what is written herein. However, by necessity there are several key terms that must be explained. I have attempted to deconstruct these explanations and include hyperlinks to certain definitions which are relevant to the subject in hand. I hope the writing generates the enthusiasm to follow up on any "oh I didn't know that" moments that may (or may not) present themselves as you read through the chapters contained in this book. The writing here is aimed at a non-specialist audience (I myself am no expert in this field), who have at least a passing interest (no matter the reason), in understanding some of what happens to the food we eat when it is digested and the power of this to change our health. The reader will come across familiar terms such as healthy living or healthy eating, but will I hope gain an appreciation of what these terms mean from a biochemical or metabolic perspective. The book is designed to inform, empower and provoke additional enthusiasm for getting back into the kitchen and take full control of your health via nutrition. As will be imparted repeatedly you do not need to reinvent the culinary wheel. In all probability you may just need to give your current wheel an extra impetus. It is hoped that the reader will be inspired to take more control over the food that they eat and maintain an interest in any future developments in the field of SIRT protein research. The essential message of this writing is to encourage further thought, discussion and provoke individual action on the role of a balanced diet on maintaining your own health. However, it is hoped that the reader gains an understanding of the systemic context in which terms such as the "obesity epidemic" are framed. Finally, this is not a book designed to preach it is a book designed to educate. So don't feel you have to read it as a novel, you can flip and skim as you see fit. Get stuck in and comments are duly welcome.

Chapter 1:
Introducing Cells, Proteins and Sirtfoods

"Our bodies are our gardens – our wills are our gardeners." William Shakespeare
Introducing Cells, Proteins and Sirtfoods

In essence a healthy metabolism means that all of your different cell types are functioning as they should. In recent years the role of Sirtfoods and Sirtuin Activators (SA's) in maintaining this healthy function has been the subject of dozens if not hundreds of individual scientific papers. The Silent Information Regulator (SIR) proteins themselves are proteins found in and around cell organelles, they exist, they are real and they are known to have a wide range of functions. This book is going to ask one fundamental question, *"Is there any credence to the notion that eating Sirtfoods can influence the activity of the SIRT proteins?"* To begin answering this question we must outline some of the biology of living cells, this will take a few sentences. Cells are the building blocks of all living organisms and the organisation of individual cells into organs and organ systems enables complete organisms to function independently in their environment. The organelles are the individual structures situated between the outer cell membrane and the inner nuclear membrane of the cell. The former membrane separates the cell contents from its external environment and controls the movement of nutrients into the cell and the removal of the waste products of metabolism. For example in respiration, oxygen and glucose are transported into the cell and the waste product carbon dioxide is removed. The nuclear membrane separates the cell cytoplasm and organelles from the nucleic acids (such as DNA) situated in the nucleus. The organelles include structures such as the mitochondria, ribosomes and Golgi apparatus. Each organelle is found in a fluid medium called the cytoplasm which is contained between the nuclear and cell membranes. Each organelle is surrounded by an exceptionally thin layer of fluid called the cytosol. The proteins themselves are a hugely diverse and absolutely essential class of biological molecules. Think of any biological or metabolic process and it is more than likely that a protein is involved. They are found in all living organisms and contain different arrangements of atoms of carbon, hydrogen, oxygen as well as nitrogen and some also contain sulphur. The term protein is derived from the Greek word *"prota"* which means *"of primary importance"*. Over two million individual proteins exist in an adult human being and each has a specific task. However, many also have additional functions.

Sirtuin proteins are known to play a crucial role in regulating biochemical process such as the cell cycle and cell reproduction. In short the SIRT proteins are widely believed to have a profound influence on metabolism in general. In biology the term *"metabolism"* refers to the totality of biochemical reactions which make life possible. At time of writing there are 7 known SIRT proteins, which are imaginatively tagged as SIRT1 to SIRT7. Without inferring any sense of priority, SIRT1 has by far been the subject of most research on the entire subject of Sirtfoods and their biochemistry. SIRT1 is widely believed to regulate the life cycles of many living cells and is also thought to influence the action of the hormone (amongst others) insulin, promote the breakdown of subcutaneous fat and regulate the tolerance to essential molecules such as glucose. At the outset it is probably helpful to impart that studies suggesting that SIRT1 as an agent of longevity have been seriously questioned by the scientific community. The subtleties pertaining to the term *"longevity"* will be addressed throughout the text and in the section hyperlinked above. Overall, the corpus of knowledge concerning Sirtfoods and the Sirt proteins themselves imparts that their activity is holistic and inter-related. When one considers their distribution within the cell, this assertion should not be surprising. Table one shows the primary location of each Sirt protein but the reader should be aware that each can be found elsewhere in the cytosol and/or cytoplasm of the cell. In addition the possible benefits are derived from studies involving laboratory animals. For example, SIRT 2 is thought to have a role in extending the life span of individual yeast cells but has to date not demonstrated an equivalent action in human beings.

Table 1 introducing the 7 (known) Sirt Compounds (Sirtuin Activators)

Name of Sirt Protein	Primary Location in the Cell	Possible metabolic Benefits
SIRT 1	Nucleus	Metabolism and respiration including promoting mitochondria formation. Enhanced brain function, alertness and cognisance.

SIRT 2	Cytosol	Unclear but is found mainly (but not exclusively) in the neurones of the brain. Possible role in mitosis and regulating aging.
SIRT 3	Mitochondria	Regulates respiration. May influence cell aging and reduce tumor formation.
SIRT 4	Mitochondria	Regulates respiration, action of insulin and fat metabolism.
SIRT 5	Mitochondria	Regulates respiration and stimulates certain enzymes. Structural repair of other Sirt proteins.
SIRT 6	Nucleus	Unknown but has strong

		correlations to controlling the symptoms of aging.
SIRT 7	Nucleus	Confirmed role in ribosome formation DNA replication and protein synthesis. May inhibit tumour formation.

Defining the SIRT proteins

SIRT1: Known to have a role in a wide range and increasing number of functions. Overall research focuses on how the compound functions and mediates in conditions which include obesity, cancer, cardiovascular and pulmonary (heart and lung) disease, dementia and stress.

SIRT2: Interest in this Sirt protein stems from the fact that it is in fact the mammalian equivalent of a protein known as Sir 2, which is found in yeast. This substance potentially has a role in tumour suppression, regulating mitosis (cell division) as well as the copying and synthesis of nucleic acids. It is thought to be a key determinant of the rate at which cells age.

SIRT3: The main focus of SIRT 3 research is its possible role as an inhibitor of tumour growth and hence is of particular interest to oncologists (scientists who study cancer). However, it may well also have a role in the stress response and so can additionally be framed as having importance in that area. Overall SIRT3 may have more importance for cancer, longevity and overall metabolic function in the male of the species.

SIRT4: Once again oncologists are interested in SIRT4 due to its apparent tumour suppressing properties. However, it also has a role in responding to nucleic acid damage, including to DNA. Researchers have additionally shown that SIRT4 regulates fatty acid oxidation in the liver and muscle cells and so could have a role in the treatment of obesity and type-2 diabetes. It is known to suppress the release of insulin from the pancreas if DNA is damaged or if the concentration of amino acids becomes too high in the blood stream. In organisms with a reduced SIRT4 level the incidence of genetic instability (mutations) increases markedly.

SIRT5: The dominant role for SIRT5 is thought to be in regulating the processes which remove ammonia and other toxins from the body via the urea cycle that is through the kidneys, renal system and liver. It is also thought to have a strong function in regulating the rate at which energy is transferred through living cells and respiration in general.

SIRT6: Perhaps underlining the importance of the sirtuins, SIRT6 is thought to be involved in the processes which govern the onset of aging. Additionally, it is known to be involved in the repair of DNA and associated structures as well as the breakdown of glucose molecules (glycolysis) and may contribute to the immune response by regulating inflammation.

SIRT7: There is a very strong body of research which indicates that SIRT7 has an important role in the transcription (copying of DNA). To complicate the work of oncologists, reduced levels of SIRT7 are known to inhibit the growth of tumors. In addition SIRT 7 may well be integral to the effective functioning, maintenance and construction of the ribosomes, which are the site of protein synthesis (manufacture) in a living cell.

A Sirtfood is any food stuff that is able to act as a source of the chemicals (nutrients from food) which stimulate Sirt protein activity. All proteins are coded for by the action of specific sequences of De-oxy Ribonucleic Acid (DNA). In other words each Sirt protein is coded for by a different gene within the molecules of DNA found in the nucleus of our cells. As can be deduced from the data presented above the precise mode of action of the sirtuins in human beings is not fully understood. However, we do know that they are enzymes and as such will be of prime importance to maintaining, regulating and otherwise influencing biochemical reactions. For example SIRT5 is known to directly control at least 700 individual proteins. From here it is fair to propose that in their entirety the sirtuins probably modulate several thousand metabolic processes. If the nucleic acids such as DNA control the biology of an organism then it may be helpful to view the sirtuins as intermediaries, in that the SIRT proteins act on the biochemical instructions passed on to them by DNA. For a food to be considered an SA it must be shown to enhance the rate at which the SIRT enzymes carry out their function. There are many thousands of individual enzymes and they all have a unique function and as a class of biological molecules they are absolutely essential to life as we know it. All enzymes accelerate the rate at which a specific biochemical (metabolic reaction) occurs, with the enzyme undergoing no chemical change in the process. Hence enzymes are often referred to as biological catalysts. For example, every single cell in every single living human being has a nucleus, except for red blood cells. In the early stages of the red blood cell cycle, the cell does possess a nucleus but over time this is substituted for the protein haemoglobin and the enzyme carbonic anhydrase. The blood vessels of the body are organised such that every single cell receives all the nutrients it needs and that all waste products are removed. In red blood cells haemoglobin carries oxygen to our approximately *forty trillion* cells and carbonic anhydrase catalyses the reaction that converts Carbon Dioxide - CO_2 (a waste product of respiration) into hydrogen carbonate. The hydrogen carbonate breaks down in the alveoli of the lungs and the CO_2 is expelled. Without carbonic anhydrase the CO_2 produced in respiration would rapidly build up becoming toxic and you would die from CO_2 poisoning very quickly indeed! In the human organism there are hundreds of different types of cell and each has a precise structure and function. Overall the thrust of research on SIRT proteins concerns their role (or not) in equally important processes and as a corollary the fundamental question asked in the opening paragraph.

The SA's are derived from various food stuffs which include leafy green vegetables such as kale, green tea and extra virgin olive oil. It gets better! If like me you are partial to a glass of vino, then you're in luck because red wine is believed to contain known SA's. Ditto if you like apple crumble, juice or its alcoholic variant, we know as cider! Furthermore, if you're partial to the occasional curry or meat, lentil or spicy bean burgers (or combinations thereof) then don't spare the turmeric. Until recently turmeric was an important dye, but was superseded by synthetic alternatives derived from the petrochemical industry. This versatile and distinctly coloured herbaceous powder has long been used in Asian cookery. Aside from providing you with quick and easy source of the compounds which are considered to be SA's, turmeric will give your food an extra boost. Not to be outdone lovers of chocolate can rest assured that a moderate intake of a high cocoa confection will boost your SA count. Finally, citrus fruits contain SA's, so instead of buying a carton of processed juice, get yourself a few oranges and squeeze them yourself. There is very little difference in cost and the taste of freshly squeezed orange juice is a different league to its concentrate derived and packaged counterpart.

Provided your diet is balanced eating foods which are high in SA's will not require any major radical change to your eating habits. For instance, I make an allowance to add kale or spinach to the sauces and soups that are regularly concocted in our kitchen. If I am making a salad then it will almost certainly have olives added and a good pokey dressing based on mustard and olive oil will be on hand for drizzling purposes. If you are making a fruit dessert or smoothie you can boost your Sirt credentials by adding blue berries and / or black currants. Having Pie and mash potato? Then add some chopped parsley with the milk, salt, pepper and mustard and work that masher as normal. If you are unsure of a side dish why not try a portion of braised greens including kale. Parsley can also be sprinkled on omelettes which from a Sirtfood perspective ought to contain olives and onions amongst the entirety of lovely fresh vegetables bound together by your mustard, pepper and herb flavoured eggs. In other words eating Sirtfoods as a normal part of a healthy balanced diet should not present most of us with any problems. In fact it would be fair to say that we are already consuming some Sirtfoods and that the only necessary point to make is that you may need to add a few more to your diet. If variety is the spice of life, then the kitchen is included, so why not experiment?

I probably shouldn't say that using fresh juices such as from black currants or red grapes to concoct your favourite tipple adds a whole new dimension to the term *"mixer"*. Oops! I've done it now; there is no going back, oh well! You better drink responsibly. In general research has yet to ascertain the precise mechanisms by which the sirtuins are activated by the chemicals present in Sirtfoods. Concurrently, it cannot as yet be categorically stated how any such activation will express itself in human beings. For example, the scientific literature contains research which asserts that the compound resveratrol may reduce the formation of the plaque in laboratory mice which have been genetically engineered to express the proteins believed to be implicated as a cause of Alzheimer's disease. The degree to which resveratrol displays the same results (if at all), has yet to be established in human suffers of Alzheimer's disease or indeed other forms of dementia such as CJD. Overall the totality of research on the efficacy of Sirt proteins on human beings (and other higher mammals) asserts that they have a non-specific and diverse range of functions. OK assuming you're still reading, let's get on with it and get things rolling by asking *"what are we talking about here?"*

Chapter 2:
What is a Sirtfood or MediterrAsian Diet?

"The Chinese do not draw a distinction between food and medicine" Lin Yutang (1895 – 1976) writing in The Importance of Living

A diet rich in Sirtfoods is also known as a (MediterrAsian) diet so named after the geographic regions in which these foods are consumed as a matter of course (the pun is 100% intended). Both Asian and Mediterranean diets are characterised by prolific consumption of fresh fish and legumes, cereals, fruit as well as non-leguminous vegetables. Dairy consumption is moderate and meat especially red meat is very low and as such the MediterrAsian diet is the complete antithesis of what is referred to in nutritional circles as the *"western diet"*. In other words the western diet is high in dairy and meat products, refined sugars and saturated fats as well as being characterised by processed and pre-packaged foods. Perhaps underlying its culinary importance the Mediterranean diet was recognised in 2013 by UNESCO as being of "intangible cultural heritage" to many Mediterranean countries. Coincidentally, in the same year, the New England Journal of Medicine published research which appears to support what we have all been told for decades. Namely, that a diet which is rich in fresh fruit and vegetables and low in fats is good for you. The above study spent 30 years following a cohort of 7,500 Spaniards aged between 55 and 85 years, split roughly equally between genders who consume the Mediterranean diet. In scientific circles it is rare to come across such succinct and direct conclusions. The interdisciplinary team of researchers state that there is an *"absolute risk reduction"* in the incidence of cardiovascular emergencies such as stroke and coronary heart disease as well as heart attacks. The research then clearly states that following the Mediterranean diet reduces the risk of such emergencies by almost a third. Without doubt this type of primary research gives empirical evidence in support of consuming a diet which is of MediterrAsian composition. It is important to stress that the researchers involved did not advocate or approve of terms such as *"superfood"*. Furthermore, there is no suggestion the diet would be a substitute for a proscribed medical treatment. In fact it was recommended to participants (in the strongest possible terms), that all such treatments should continue. However, in terms of a preventative measure that can be easily integrated into a person's lifestyle choices the evidence is more than compelling. In fact too many people think such findings represent a succinct definition of the term *"self-evident"*.

In this particular study weight loss or longevity were not the subjects of study and individuals were not given strict menu regimes or generally required to count the calories. In short participants were allowed a bit of *"what they fancy"* as long as they kept to the overall dietary requirements necessary to participate in the study. In the world of Sirtfoods you are not sticking to a strict dietary regime with an equally punishing exercise schedule. You are following a healthy balanced diet plus a few necessary extras, washed down by the occasional treat. In this particular study only 7% of participants dropped out within two years but in contrast 14% of people dropped out in the part of the study where diet was much more proscriptive. This is good news because it should impart that anyone can follow a diet rich in Sirtfoods provided they make a little effort and of course keep improving their cooking skills. The research did acknowledge the cost of certain ingredients such as extra virgin oil which does cost more than other types of olive oil. The difference isn't much, but if you're on a budget every penny counts and so in the real world cost is a factor.

Whether they intended to or not, to acknowledge this fact the scientists involved provided participants with extra virgin oil and any other ingredients as necessary to keep them on board. Having stated that, it is equally important to stress that the foods mentioned below are affordable, have proven nutritional benefits and are easy to incorporate into your diet if you are spending time in the kitchen; that is not just at parties. The next section provides an overview of the principle Sirtfoods, their vitamin and mineral content as well as any information pertaining to the SIRT proteins the food may activate. It is important to realise that the properties outlined below are not an exhaustive list and the reader is encouraged to follow up on any stand of information presented as they see fit. The reader should also be aware that many of the substances discussed are present in more than one food. Finally, the benefits presented below should be viewed from a perspective where the person is not undergoing any prescribed medical treatment. The points made should only impart that eating these food stuffs can be easily integrated into any balanced diet and are in no way a substitute for advice from your doctor or dietitian.

Black Currants and Blue Berries:

Aside from tasting absolutely incredible blue berries are a rich source of polyphenol compounds, the particular type being named anthocyanin. Now, you do not need to know the precise chemical structure or even make up of this family of organic (carbon based) chemicals. You do need to appreciate that polyphenols are highly efficient anti-oxidants and so help the cell resist damage from what is termed Cellular Oxidative Stress (COS), which is outlined in the section on **free radicals.** Anthocyanin has been shown to protect laboratory animals from neurological damage and improve their cognitive functions. In clinical (human) trials anthocyanin has been shown to improve the memory function of older adults suffering from dementia. Further research imparts that a preventative function for anthocyanin is more likely if food stuffs such as blueberries are consumed regularly and as part of a normal balanced diet. Overall blue berries are a high density source of anti-oxidants, vitamins such as A, C, and E as well as essential trace elements such as selenium, potassium, copper, iron and manganese. Blue berries are an important source of the B vitamins which are known to facilitate the metabolism of the three principle types of biological molecules (fats, proteins and carbohydrates). Ok so you get the point, blue berries are good. In terms of SIRT protein research continues but the anti-oxidants present are thought to promote the action of SIRT1 and SIRT 2. In general terms black currants are believed to express equivalent health benefits.

Green Tea:

Green tea is native to India and China where its health benefits have been recognised for centuries, it is the unrefined form of the more familiar black tea and accounts of about 20% of all the tea that is consumed globally. Green tea is well known to contain more anti-oxidants, such as polyphenols than its black and more processed counterpart. For example a polyphenol known as epigallocatechin-3-gallate (EGCG) is according to some medical researchers the polyphenol most associated with preventing the incidence of tumours. Helpfully ECGC is one of many key active polyphenols in green tea. A cursory google search will present the corpus of knowledge that indicates a chemo-preventative role for ECGC in laboratory animals and it may even help the body cope with chemotherapy. In addition epidemiological (people) studies have shown some reduction in the risk of cancers of the stomach, colon, blood vessels, skin, prostate gland, bladder, lungs, the breasts (mammary glands) and oesophagus. In terms of cancer prevention ECGC is thought to function by suppressing the factors which allow cancer cells to develop in the first instance. Overall medical research suggests that ECGC has great potential for the treatment of disease, particularly cancer in homo-sapiens this should not be surprising due to the pedigree which the green tea plant possesses. In traditional medicines green tea leaves are used to treat wounds, improve the functioning of the heart and mental faculties and in the diet it is known to help digestion, it may even help with thermo-regulation (science speak for maintaining an optimum body temperature). In terms of biology of the Sirtuin proteins, green tea is believed to stimulate the proteins involved in metabolism and may contribute to effective treatment for type-2 diabetes. Additionally, green tea is known to contain *"anti-inflammatory agents"* and could very well promote the activity of all 7 Sirt proteins. Green tea is also a rich source of vitamin K, folic acid and Fluoride.

Dark Chocolate And Cocoa:

Right, shall we get something straight right away; the health benefits outlined here are not meant to signal that you can go to the nearest corner shop and gorge yourself on processed chocolate. We are talking here about a cocoa content and put simply the purported health benefits apply more to the cocoa beans themselves and not to the confection. So seek out high cocoa content chocolate that exceeds 70%, contains no refined sugar, few if any additives or added fats. Limited research exists which implies that cocoa may reduce blood pressure and therefore may have a role treating hypertension as well as maintaining a healthy cardiovascular system. However, this is by no means a certainty and the same can be said for research which suggests cocoa may have a role in preventing bowel (colon) cancer. There are equivalently strong research findings which suggest that cocoa may inhibit the action of stress hormones, but once again the actual scientific basis for the assertion is far from being established. However, the presence of compounds known as flavonoids which are another class of organic compounds related to the poly phenols, implies effective anti-oxidant properties. The flavonoids are also present in green tea, black tea, fruits, berries and thankfully red wine, so cheers! In its totality unrefined cocoa beans contain over 400 biologically active chemicals amongst them is the amino acid tryptophan. At this juncture I'm afraid we need to introduce some more biology!

In total there are 20 amino acids and they are the building blocks for all the proteins in existence. All of the two million (or thereabouts) proteins in the human body and the millions more which exist across the biosphere are made from the same 20 amino acids. Each protein is made (synthesised) in the cell organelle we name the ribosome. The really clever part is that our DNA ensures that each protein is made with an exact and precise order of amino acids, but the not so clever part is that human beings (along with other species of mammal) need to ingest the amino acids we need to manufacture proteins. We acquire these amino acids from proteins, which must first be eaten and digested. In other words the amino acids we use to synthesise proteins were (whether plant or animal) once part of the protein structure of another organism. Tryptophan has an affinity for an enzyme called tryptophan hydrolase which helps assemble tryptophan into the neurotransmitter (substance which transfers nerve signals from one nerve cell to another) serotonin (amongst others). Hence it follows that amino acids are essential for the effective functioning of the brain and from here we can impart that effective protein synthesis is dependent on healthy ribosomes. If the SIRT proteins in their entirety are essential for healthy metabolism then it may be established that for SIRT7 to be effective on the ribosomes, the other SIRT proteins must have the metabolic conditions in which to function effectively. It is entirely possible that any number of the active chemicals contained within cocoa beans could well be SA's, however it cannot be stressed enough, that this notion is far from being demonstrated. For now enjoy real chocolate as part of a healthy living program and remember that you just don't know what future benefits may present themselves.

Olives and Extra Virgin Olive Oil:

Arguably, the food most associated with the Mediterranean region is the green and black oval shaped fruit from the *Olea Europaea* tree. Since the time of Ancient Greece the olive tree has been the symbol of peace and cooperation because the substances contained in the fruit and the oils derived from it are so essential to a diet built around healthy living. As such the *O.Europea* tree has been valued for thousands of years both as a store of energy in the form of essential fats and for its high concentration of anti-oxidants. Olives are the source of oleocanthal and oleurpein which are recognised as very powerful natural anti-oxidants and along with high concentrations of carotenoids are certainly wonderful drops of good stuff, which may additionally help the body combat diseases ranging from cancer to diabetes to dementia. However, it is unlikely that terms such as "*anti-oxidant*" were used to describe their importance until comparatively recently, I mean oxygen wasn't even discovered until the late 18th century, well 1774 to be precise! Olives contain mono unsaturated fats such as oleic and palmitoleic acid which is known to lower levels of a molecules termed low density lipo-proteins (LDL). At this juncture it is crucial that the reader understands that despite the bad press cholesterol is actually essential for healthy metabolism. It is synthesised in the liver and ingested via the consumption of animal fats, in the body cholesterol is used in the manufacture of hormones, aids in the stability of the cell membrane. In digestion enzymes in the liver convert cholesterol into some of the acidic substances which make up bile an important digestive fluid stored in the gall bladder. As part of the digestive process fats are broken in the ileum which is the later part of the small intestine, where fats are emulsified. In essence, bile is secreted from the gall bladder into the ileum and the fats are mechanically broken down into smaller droplets. Emulsification of fats provides a larger surface area upon which the lipase enzymes can catalyse the reactions which break down fats into fatty acids. When this process finishes the bile acids are absorbed back into the blood stream and transported back to the glass bladder and re-used. In short the body does not need very much if any extra cholesterol, it can manufacture enough from the food we eat. Hence if you are eating too much animal fat cholesterol can build up in the blood stream and so the LDL's come into play and carry to sites of deposition, which include but are not limited to the walls of the arteries. In general terms the more cholesterol being carried and deposited by LDL's the greater is the likelihood of serious trauma such as a heart attack. In contrast High Density Lipo-proteins (HDL) work in the opposite direction that is they carry cholesterol from sites of deposition to the liver, where it is broken down into soluble substances and any waste products expelled. Any food such as olives and extra virgin oil which is rich in mono-unsaturated fats promotes the action of HDL's over that of LDL's hence reducing the probability of Atherosclerosis and of suffering from heart attack induced by Coronary Heart Disease (CHD).

The oils contained within the (not so) humble olive also have anti-inflammatory properties and themselves contain high concentrations of vitamin E (alpha-tocopherol), which is lipid (fat) soluble and plays a crucially important role in holding cell membranes together. Vitamin E also has a role in the free radical clean up discussed below. Just in case you weren't feeling healthy enough olives also contain plenty of trace metallic elements such as zinc, calcium, copper, iron and manganese as well as a smattering of B vitamins including niacin, pantothenic acid and choline. Finally, I am always arguing with my wonderful girlfriend on the virtues of purchasing "*extra virgin*" as opposed to "*olive oil*". The former is cold pressed and so loses none of the nutrients and essential substances discussed above, more importantly it comes as nature intended because to meet the designation "extra virgin" it must not be processed in anyway shape or form. In terms of Sirtuin Activation the substances locked up inside both green and black olives could promote the action of any Sirt protein involved in regulating anti-oxidant activity, respiration and mitochondrial function, influencing the onset of the symptoms of ageing as well as the rate of fatty acid breakdown.

Kale:

Although phrases such as "superfood" ought to be taken with the proverbial pinch of salt kale would certainly fit into the category. Kale of one type or another has been eaten for thousands of years. This nutritionally dense leafy green vegetable contains vitamins A, K and C as well as trace minerals including manganese and potassium (amongst others), in short you could do very well in the healthy living stakes by eating kale on a regular basis. Kale also contains many of the B vitamins as well as non–metallic elements such as phosphorus. As if that wasn't good enough kale is also an important source of linoleic acid, which is one of the omega-3 fatty acids and all of this is combined with a very low calorie count. Kale continues to get better, as it has a very high concentration of the anti-oxidants which belong to both the polyphenol and flavonoid classes of organic compounds. The two principle flavonoids are the compounds quercetin and kaempferol, but taken together the anti-oxidant credentials of Kale means that it may have essential role in promoting cardiovascular health, reducing blood pressure as well as being anti-inflammatory, anti-viral and it may have role in suppressing the spread and growth of tumours. The kale plant contains substances such as sulforaphane and many others which have been shown to inhibit the growth and spread (metastasis) of cancer cells in laboratory animals; however, there is no clear cut evidence of the same processes occurring in human beings. In terms of the reduction of cardiovascular disease kale has the same broad spectrum of benefits concerning the lowering of LDL's as the fats contained within olives and cold pressed olive oil.

Now then! Here is another idea for your kitchen, steam your vegetables! The reason is simple if you boil for too long many of the nutrients will pass out into the water, I mean why else does it take on the colour of the food you are cooking. I suppose you can keep the cooking water as stock, but if you steam significantly less nutrient loss occurs in the first place. Hence, steaming vegetables means more lovely nutrients with long unpronounceable names will be able to fulfil their function in your body as compared to boiling them. In terms of its Sirt credentials kale contains many of the chemical families that have been associated with the efficacy of SIRT proteins so it seems reasonable to postulate that in general terms eating kale could be beneficial. However, more research will be needed before any definite association can be asserted. One area of research is the relationship between sulforaphane and the mechanisms by which it stimulates the enzymes which break down carcinogens.

(Useful video) http://nutritionfacts.org/video/second-strategy-to-cooking-broccoli

Parsley:

Parsley is native to the Mediterranean and has been used for thousands of years as both a herbal medicine and as an accompaniment which improves the flavour and aesthetics of many dishes. The scientific name of the herb is *Petroselinum crispum* and has been confused with coriander more times than I care to mention. It is now used all over the world and is rich source of Vitamin K, C and A in addition to the anti-oxidants outlined elsewhere in this chapter. One of the anti-oxidants present in parsley is a flavonol called Myricetin which has been shown to have demonstrable chemo-preventative impact on skin cancer. The term chemo prevention refers to any therapy or prophylactic (preventative treatment) that uses naturally occurring (normally plant based) compounds or their manufactured counterparts to prevent or treat a cancer. At this juncture it is important to note that the medical professionals in the field do not consider cancer to be a single disease. According Cancer Research UK over 200 different types of cancer have been diagnosed and each has a different and precise mode of action. In the world of cancer research and treatment the role of diet in cancer prevention is receiving more and intense scrutiny from those who are seeking to cure this terrifying disease. Other foods which contain high levels of Myricetin include sweet potatoes, black currants and cranberries. Myricetin is also of interest to those scientists interested in the treatment of type 2 diabetes because of its potential in promoting insulin activity (i.e. the formation of glycogen). In terms of Sirt activation parsley contains many of the substances that are discussed elsewhere in this section and the same can be said for the other recognised Sirtfoods.

these foods contain to varying degrees the vitamins
and other substances which are thought to be involve
protein activation. Some SA's will be present
concentrations in one food as compared to and
example, we cannot categorically state that Miso so
its variants) is a greater SIRT protein activator
turmeric because we simply do not know. However
expanding amount of research on the subject it
matter of time before such assertions will be made.
will this take? Well how long is a piece of string? 1
should not see this as an issue or stumbling block, ir
the opposite. Suppose it was established that M
activated SIRT7 and turmeric or loveage activate
There is no problem here all you would do is add s
to your soup as a garnish and perhaps add turme
risotto you are having for your main evening meal
night. Said Risotto should also contain onions, pars
served with a salad rich in olives and drizzled with e
olive oil. As will be said again and again and
keyword is balance. The essential point of this cha
make clear that it is not necessary to partake
supplements (unless you have been advised to do s
doctor). Furthermore, the reader should conclude
these foods have a preventative role in mitigating
ranging from diabetes to cancer, they are not cures.
in terms of healthy living there is no substitute
control of your diet and that means informing and
yourself. In a very real sense this chapter should be v
signpost to healthy eating habits. So, to answer th
titular question a Sirtfood diet is one which encou
take control of what you are eating and how you

food. It allows you to add a wide range of readily available ingredients to your diet in a creative and interesting way. It enables you to tick all of your nutritional boxes without breaking the bank. It means you can cook amazing food for yourself, friends, family and loved ones quickly as well as improving and expanding your culinary expertise. Oh and it could well improve your biochemistry and keep you out of hospital for a few more years, which sounds like a plan to me! In its entirety, ingesting Sirtfoods dovetails with eminent synergy to notions of following a balanced diet. Unfortunately, it is not as easy as it sounds just to add some olives or fresh vegetables to your diet if your circumstances do not allow it. It is true that millions of people are regularly consuming the Sirtfoods discussed above, but significant numbers of people in the UK are not and the next chapter will attempt to provide an overview as to why this is the case.

Chapter 3:
Calorie Restriction and Sirtuin Activation

"A long healthy life is no accident. It begins with good genes, but it also depends on good habits" Dan Buettner (explorer and endurance athlete)

Calorific Restriction (CR) as a mechanism by which to improve metabolism as part of what we would now term a balanced Plant based or Mediterr-Asian diet, is not a new undertaking. In terms of improved lifespan and quality of life the possible benefits of CR have been known since the 1930's. However, the idea that the SIRT proteins could improve these effects was established at around the year 2000. As such there is a long way to go before any definite assertions can be made. What can be said is that in laboratory animals different sirtuins have different effects on the physiology of the animals. From here it is fair to say that the potential for metabolic benefits derived from Sirtuin Activation (SA) could be augmented under conditions of a regulated CR diet. As of 2015 human trials have not been carried out and many of the experiments undertaken in the laboratory have been with genetically engineered animals. In other words these experiments were not carried out it in "real world" and are at this stage indicators of a potential (but likely) positive metabolic impact. Aside from these points the point is that the SIRT proteins can have enhanced metabolic impacts and will likely have long term benefits for the physiology and metabolism of mammals including human beings. Furthermore as has been made abundantly clear in this book a balanced and varied diet is a sure fire way to ingest the entirety of sirtuin activating chemicals. Hence once again there is no reason not to expand your diet irrespective of the writing presented below.

Specific chemicals present in the Mediterr-Asian diet such as resveratrol derived from red wine or oleuropein and hydroxytyrosol from olive oil and isoflavones from soybeans and ECGC are known to activate SIR1 proteins. Given the suggested roles of SIR1 in human metabolism some food scientists suggest that CR may increase this particular mode of action. From this position it is not unrealistic to infer that as part of a balanced diet and / or modulated dietary regimen that calorie restriction may boost the activation of all seven sirtuin proteins. One strand in the area of CR and SA concerns the hypothesised inhibition of serious health conditions such as Coronary Heart Disease CHD and Cardio Vascular Disease (CVD), type 2 diabetes, neurological disease as well as some forms of cancer. Additionally and irrespective of the actual mechanisms at work it appears that CR and the eating of polyphenol containing foodstuffs could have similar metabolic impacts on human beings. Furthermore a principle mechanism by which food derived polyphenols have their function amplified is through SA biochemistry. CR refers to a strict dietary protocol where the diet is reduced by any quantity up to 40%. When applied to micro-organism such as yeast, the glucose was cut by 40%, the budding lifespan of the yeast was significantly extended. It is not surprising that experimental findings such as these encourage interest in CR both as a method of extending quality and length of life in mammals. Research continues apace and findings continue to be contradictory, reflecting the complexity of the science being undertaken. For example, some studies suggest that the presence of yeast SIR2 is responsible for the increase in budding lifespan, others that its presence has no effect on reproduction. CR is a regimen that will have different impacts on different organs and therefore the entire human organism and these effects will vary between individuals. Hence there is no one size fits all approach and CR itself remains a deeply emotive area of research. As will be stressed again toward the end of this chapter it should only be carried out under the guidance of health care professionals. For our purposes there is a very real possibility that the activity of the sirtuins themselves may be augmented under the metabolic conditions induced by a CR regimen. In other words as the BMI (Body Mass Index) is reduced under the auspices of a Mediterr-Asian or Plant Based Diet (PBD) the very real benefits of Sirt Protein biochemistry are augmented.

The essential basis of CR is that it reduces levels of undesirable fats and LDL cholesterol (amongst other substances) in the blood stream as well as keeping the blood pressure within optimal homeostatic limits. All of these variables are implicated in both Coronary Heart Disease (CHD) and Cardio Vascular Disease (CVD). Furthermore the hormones leptin as indicated in chapter five and adiponectin in chapter 6 are key indicators of metabolic imbalance as expressed by their interaction with the hypothalamus. As numbers of adipose (fat) cells are steadily reduced leptin levels are reduced whilst those of adiponectin are increased and the appetite becomes balanced such that the person experiences the feeling of being "full" after they have eaten less food. Furthermore because adiponectin expresses anti-inflammatory, anti-atherogenic, insulin activity properties, it is highly likely to be protective against CVD and help with the treatment of type-2 diabetes.

Chapter two introduced the term "oxidative stress" and as we age our cells become more susceptible to its ravages. As biological molecules and organelles age they repair less readily and begin to accumulate in the cellular environment. Concurrently, the anti-oxidant capabilities of the body progressively degrade as we get older. In addition a perfect biologically negative storm arises as our metabolism changes because the production of ROS is widely to considered to increase in our later years. It is important to reiterate that the creation of ROS is a normal part of healthy metabolism and that the charged particles are not some sort of metabolic bogey man. At low concentrations ROS are known to benefit cellular processes in addition because the ROS cause a response at a molecular level in mammals (including ourselves) they induce adaptive effects which may well lead to new evolutionary pathways. As a whole ROS substances may garner long term benefit by acting as signalling molecules which could regulate the REDOX processes outlined in chapter 6. A managed program of CR could enhance such processes because when the body is not receiving new inputs of the metabolites of carbohydrate and fat digestion, more ROS species are produced when energy reserves are broken down.

SIRT 1 is often viewed as the gate keeper sirtuin against molecular and cellular oxidative stress as well as a protector against damage to nucleic acids, including DNA. During experiments on cell cultures researchers have demonstrated that during conditions of simulated CR that mammalian SIR1 activity is enhanced in the muscles, brain, kidneys and in adipose cells. The result as demonstrated by the experiments is that under conditions of CR numbers of adipose cells progressively decrease and as this occurs the body becomes more sensitive to the action of insulin. Intertwined with such a notion is research which suggests that under these circumstances SIRT 1 also promotes the action of those genes which promote glucose formation in the liver as opposed to that of glycogen. Simultaneously, SIRT 1 promotes the breakdown of fatty acids in the cell mitochondria. In the pancreas of laboratory animals the activation of SIRT 1 under conditions of CR promotes the increase of insulin and therefore breaks up of glycogen and fatty acids into glucose. At the same time the SIRT proteins in general are believed to protect the liver and other organs against the oxidative stress produced by changes in metabolism.

Having said all of this there is contradictory data concerning all of these suppositions such that there is equally robust research which suggests that under conditions of CR that the activity of all sirt proteins can be suppressed and may even elicit the opposite metabolic effects, such that fat is more readily synthesised and accumulated. However, these findings tend to be the result of feeding laboratory animals the equivalent of a human western diet. To further complicate matters different species of rodents expressed varying degrees of metabolic change. However, some of the discrepancy can be explained by diet such that the more fat (in particular saturated fat) the less effective where the SIRT proteins in general and SIRT 1 in particular. From this it is tentatively possible to suggest that a low fat diet promotes sirtuin activity and that for this activity to be most effective the diet itself must be balanced. In other words for the sirtuins to be effective the person must have balanced metabolism as indicated by an appropriate BMI. By definition a principle reason for embarking on any kind of CR is to lose weight and reduce the harm that a western diet causes to the circulatory system in particular and the rest of the body in general. Cardiovascular disease (CVD) is a huge killer and is characterised by high levels of LDL cholesterol, hardened and plaqued arteries (arthrosclerosis). Unsurprisingly in countries where the Western diet is the general norm CVD is a huge killer. According to the WHO CVD is the biggest cause of death across the world, accounting for over 30% of global mortality in 2012. During a regimen of CR SIR1 has been shown to inhibit inflammation and has been associated with decreased levels of both adipose tissue and cholesterol. Furthermore under these conditions the ability of the human body to excrete cholesterol and fat appear to be enhanced.

It is well understood that a degree of exercise is essential for healthy metabolism. In the human body there are various enzymes which are widely believed to activate the 7 sirtuin proteins. Science has yet to establish the precise mode of action of these relationships but strong indicators exist that in times of high energy expenditure and low energy inputs that energy sensing enzymes and cell signalling molecules have mutually beneficial synergistic relationship. In other words the sirtuin proteins are more active because they have stimulated to do so when the body is "burning off" its reserves of energy (i.e. fat cells). The research literature further implies that such responses are a normal physiological response to an increase in demand for chemical energy (i.e. from respiration). In addition it appears that during times of CR and other mechanisms of achieving metabolic balance that the process of autogaphy discussed in chapter six is enhanced. SIR1 is by far the most studies of the sirtuin proteins but as chapter one makes clear it is not the only one (pun intended). For example the efficacy sirtuins 3 and 4 promoted during times of CR, this is crucial because SIR3 is expressed in the brain, liver and kidneys and in a specific type of adipose tissue known as brown fat cells. One function of these cells is to act as an energy source in new born infants with the express purpose of generating the heat needed to maintain the body temperature at 37°C. As SIR3 is expressed that is brown fat cells are metabolised more rapidly, the activity of SIR4 is inhibited. This inhibition by series of exceptionally complex biochemical pathways (that we are far from fully understanding) stimulates the production of insulin and so could have utility in the treatment of diabetes.

All of this should give the reader the impression that the active compounds that are derived from a Mediterr-Asian and PBD do not act in isolation from each other. There are clear and definite relationships between these substances which collectively have a role in keeping the metabolism in balance and therefore the person healthier for a longer a period of time. A CR should never be attempted off the cuff that is without the consent of a health professional. It is simply not possible to maintain a full CR diet for long periods of time without undergoing significant tissue and organ wastage as well as reductions in everything from libido to cognitive function. If advised and under a properly controlled dietary regimen which is rich in the Sirtfoods discussed throughout this book, then a preventative and potential reversing effect may express itself. However, this is by no means guaranteed and CR still remains a highly emotive and controversial subject.

In 2013 researchers at the University of Washington established a mechanism by which SIR1 operates in the brain under periods of CR. In this example the research team showed that CR enhanced the activity of SIR1 on the hypothalamus (see chapter four) promoting increased activity inside the bones and muscles (the musculoskeletal system). The research is based on findings from experiments carried out on laboratory animals that had been genetically engineered to over express SIR1 in certain organs. The animals where fed a normal rodent diet and those that expressed the SIR1 in the brain were found to have improved musculoskeletal function. In addition the sleep pattern of this cohort of animals was much more regular than their peers; furthermore, this was associated with better temperature regulation and much more regular rates of respiration. Overall this cohort of mice lived longer, was healthier and was much less likely to develop disease, preventable or otherwise. It is crucially important to impart that such research does not suggest that CR and SIRT activation mean that animals live longer. The researchers in this study are quick to state that the onset of ageing is postponed but not its pace, such that ageing and the potential for developing age related diseases is delayed but not stopped. In other words one day you are still going to depart this mortal coil, no matter how healthy you are. You are mortal deal with it! Having said that, the scientist involved have identified the parts of the hypothalamus and the specific genes that activate this segment of SIR1 biochemistry. The increase in signalling facilitated by SIR1 in the hypothalamus could prove to have significant implications for the prevention and treatment of the diseases associated with ageing. Intertwined with such findings is the knowledge that in experiments on insects and other arthropods and even yeast, a direct and positive relationship between SIR2 and ageing is clear and apparent. In other words those organisms with SIR2 in their adipose cells lived longer than those which did not.

In short as the remainder of this book will impart there is years of research ahead for those scientists in the field of nutrition and sirtuin biochemistry. However, a very solid foundation exists which sets the scene for further strong indicators of a causative connection between SA and CR in particular as well as diet in general. Such that the more foods which are known to contain SA's are eaten the more likely that the Sirt proteins will be activated, function together synergistically and holistically, to the overall benefit of our physiology.

Chapter 4:
Perspectives on Malnutrition

"The best doctors give the least medicine" Benjamin Franklin

It cannot be overstated that the nutritional benefits of consuming Sirtfoods will only present themselves if you are consuming a balanced diet. Any high school biology text book will impart that to be balanced a diet must provide all of the nutrients in the correct amounts which allow the human organism to carry out its seven life processes. Malnutrition is generally associated with a situation in which people are not consuming enough of any of the principle food groups. These groups in their entirety contain the carbohydrates, fats, proteins as well as the vitamins, minerals, water and dietary roughage necessary for healthy living. Malnutrition is generally associated to situations where the organism has no alternative but to first breakdown its reserves of glycogen and then fats. This metabolism provides the energy needed to keep the body functioning but does not replace nutrients. The only mechanism by which mammals including human beings can replenish their stock of nutrients is by eating. Thus, if our nutrient reserves are not replaced by feeding the body will start to break down tissues such as muscle to stay alive. We understand this occurrance as starvation and it currently affects according to the UN Food and Agricultural organisation (UNFAO) approximately 800 million people globally. Far from being curtailed such instances of malnutrition are now increasingly occurring in the more prosperous countries.

Until the onset of the crisis and austerity economics it would have been fair to state that in the Western world access to and the affordability of food was overall not an issue. Irrespective of your income or social class most of us could afford to consume a balanced diet. When one considers the reality of food banks in the UK alone, it is equally fair to state that the above pronouncement no longer holds true. According to the Trussel Trust (a charity which seeks to end food poverty in the UK) over 1 million people are given weekly emergency food parcels to prevent the malnutrition we generally associate with the Global South (i.e. majority world). The picture across continental Europe is equally stark. According to the European Federation of Food Banks (EFFB) across the European Union (EU) over 125 million people are experiencing some degree of food poverty. Even the more affluent European countries such as Norway have now set up food banks to feed people who can no longer afford to purchase enough to eat. At time of writing Oslo has the dubious honour of being the location for the EFFB's 257th European food bank. Unfortunately, these numbers look set to increase. Such is the negative impacts of cuts on the overall health of any nation, with the poor and most vulnerable members of society suffering disproportionately. Across the Atlantic Ocean US based NGO "Hunger Notes", asserts that almost 15% of all U.S households are experiencing food poverty. Put simply food poverty is a situation where people have to make an invidious choice between eating or heating, or feeding their children but not themselves. As of 2015 the number of people experience food poverty in the UK continues to rise. However, overall in parts of the world where the so called "western diet" is the norm an opposite form of malnutrition occurs. Instead of starving malnourished people in the Western world tend to be overweight or obese. These populations do not generally experience Kwashiorkor (protein deficiency) but do have an increased incidence of Type 2 diabetes, cardiovascular disease (stroke, heart attack, and atherosclerosis) as well as disorders to the skeletal system and even some forms of cancer. The consequences of the availability of cheap processed food which is high in fat, refined sugar and salt, whilst simultaneously being low in fibre, vitamins and minerals are clear and present. According to the WORLD HEALTH ORGANISATION a minimum of 2.8 million people are killed globally every year because of complications resulting from obesity. In the UK the figure is approximately 6% of the overall death rate which translates very roughly into several thousand deaths per year as of 2014. In short you can rest assured that if a population is not consuming its recommended 5 a day, then it certainly isn't getting its daily quota of Sirtfoods. Again it must be stressed, that Sirtfoods are not some wonder superfood; they are essential components of a balanced diet. As such they should be made available to all under the auspices of initiatives such as the Food for Life Partnership (FFLP).

It is undeniable that the global population is experiencing a profound obesity problem. Or more precisely the countries whose populations consume *"the western diet"* are experiencing a profound obesity problem. The word "obesity" is deceptively simple and the study of its causes and consequences spans across the major disciplines of the social, biological and chemical sciences. Thus, to answer the question *"what causes obesity?"* requires a holistic and considered response. At its most basic level obesity is a result of a convergence of the availability and consumption of foods which are processed and nutrient deficient in combination with a lack of regular exercise. Things become more complex when the relative availability and perceived affordability of so called *"junk food"* is compared to that of *"real food"*. A key thrust of this book is to state that integrating Sirtfoods (most of which already have established healthy eating benefits), should not be an issue provided you have access to them and can afford to buy them. Sadly, in modern Britain access to fresh wholesome and healthy food has become an issue for many communities. For instance, consider the reality of food deserts, a term which has entered popular parlance over the twenty years from 1995 to the present day. In the proverbial nutshell most people are aware of the health benefits of fresh fruit and vegetables. However, what happens if the community contains no outlets for any of the foods that are considered to be healthy or even worse people simply cannot afford to buy it. In such a context the nearest frozen food retailer or take away shop is going to be a much more attractive and convenient option. A food desert is loosely defined as any region where no reliable and affordable outlet for fresh fruit and vegetables exists within a set distance (anywhere up to 1000m) from a given residential community.

As of 2015 the number of food deserts in the UK is thought to several dozen and their existence is directly associated with dietary issues which fall under the term obesity. It is beyond the scope of this book to examine the causes of the wholly undesirable food desert phenomenon but their prevalence is correlated with the development of out of town supermarkets and the cutting back of essential public services, such as transport. Additionally, the phenomenon is not limited to the UK and it is not just a question of access. It is also a question of affordability and education. Over the years I've spoken to many of the younger generation who cannot tell the difference between different fruits and vegetables and many who have never opened up a cook book before or who even have a regular home prepared meal. In addition many of these children have answered *"from the supermarket"* when asked the question *"where does our food come from?"* These were not quintessentially deprived inner city children who had never seen a tree outside of a park before, but privileged

European students in fee paying schools. I can categorically state that a lack of education around food does not respect social class. Additionally, I remember being taught at school and at home how to boil an egg or how to make different sauces. In my last year of secondary school we had "*survival cookery*" classes' last thing on Friday afternoons. I learnt how to make pasta, rice, pizza bases, bread and burgers (from scratch) as well dishes such as risotto. To my knowledge there is no commitment on any school (due to a lack of funding as opposed to intent) to offer home economics or domestic science (cooking) classes to their students. Without doubt this and other factors concerning our "*connection to the food eat*" are contributors to the current dire situation.

As the 21st century progresses the number of obesity related deaths all over the Western world continues its annual increase. According to the World Health Organisation (WHO) obesity across the board has doubled over the 35 years since 1980. The figures speak for themselves; in 1980 approximately 800 million people were diagnosed as being clinically obese. At time of writing the WHO estimates that approximately one third of the entire population (two billion people) are overweight and that 10% are clinically obese. Furthermore, a staggering 42 million children under 5 can now be categorised as overweight or obese. To make matters worse the numbers are actually increasing, such that by 2030 predictions of billions of people being obese (as opposed to merely being overweight) are not unusual. The truly shocking fact is that over half of this number lives in just 10 countries. The UK is likely to join this wholly undesirable club in a few short years. According to research published in the UK as of 2014, over half of women and close two thirds of men are overweight or obese. Furthermore, suggestions that half of the population of the UK will be obese by 2050 are not unrealistic assertions.

The next chapter will look at how Sirtfoods can mitigate this form of malnutrition.

Chapter 5:
Why are Sirtfoods so Beneficial?

"The doctor of the future will no longer treat the human frame with drugs, but rather will cure and prevent disease with nutrition." Thomas Edison

It is suffice to impart that being "overweight" and being "obese" are different extremes of the same eating disorder. Irrespective of the cause obesity occurs when you consume more food and calories than your body needs to fulfill its energetic and life processing requirements. Any excess food is converted to fat which is then stored subcutaneously in the legs and abdomen. In other words obesity is a consequence of feeding more than metabolising. The fat in an obese person has accumulated to such an extent that healthy living and normal metabolic function is impaired. It is absolutely beyond the remit of this writing to explore in any great detail the social consequences of the sorry state of affairs outlined in the previous chapter. However, it is possible to extract several key factors and intimate how implementing a Sirtfood and balanced diet can reduce the social and economic consequences which are inextricably bound up in terms such as "*global obesity epidemic*".

The most familiar method by which we define the terms overweight and obese is by use of a simple mathematical function we know as the Body Mass Index (BMI). Whilst there are several issues with the methodology concerning BMI calculations, the health impacts of being obese are clear and present.

The calculation is very simple:

Body Mass in Kg / Height in Metres = BMI

The World Health Organisation (WHO) defines an obese person as having a BMI of more than 30 and you are overweight if your BMI exceeds 25. In extreme cases a BMI of over 40 delimits, chronic and potentially life threatening severe obesity. The numerical outcome of this simple equation is used to establish a base line from which to ascertain the broad strokes concerning an individual's eating habits. In other words the BMI is not a diagnosis of obesity it is an indicator. However, to be distracted by this fact is to take the next left turn to the confused town known as semantics, the economic alone cost is staggering. For example research published by the McKinsey Global Institute (a global management consultancy) in November 2014 outlines the reasons why obesity costs the UK economy some £47 Billion per year, which translates to a loss of 3% in GDP. Globally the MGI report states that obesity constitutes 5% of the global death rate and a loss of approximately $2 trillion, which is about 3% of GDP.

The social cost to the UK in terms of NHS treatment for conditions such as stroke, type 2 diabetes, Cardiovascular conditions, breast and colon cancer as well as a whole host of other ailments is calculated to be about £6 billion per year, currently the UK spends around 1% on obesity prevention programmes. On top of this huge figure an additional £10 billion is spent on treatment for diabetes related to obesity. In other words £16 billion is spent annually on treating conditions that are by and large preventable. To put things into perspective the total financial commitment to dealing with obesity is more than is spent on the police, probation, law courts and fire brigade, combined. The MGI report suggests that if nothing is done then by 2030 the figure for treating obesity (excluding type 2 diabetes) alone could balloon to £12 billion; by any benchmark this is clearly unacceptable. Overall, the MGI report recommends a coordinated response to the problem; such a response includes nutritional education and provision of healthy school and work place meals, which are affordable for all, the parallels with FFLP should be obvious. It advocates a school curriculum which integrates exercise and domestic science. It sees the benefits of the provision of facilities ranging from more cycle lanes to subsidised membership for gyms and health clubs. The report contains many other excellent suggestions and solutions which are aimed at individuals and communities, but also says that funding for such initiatives is essential. All of these initiatives have the capacity to help and to quote the director of the MGI *"Efforts to address obesity have been piecemeal up till now. Yet obesity is a systemic issue, born of many interlocking factors, and only a systemic response will do."* I could not have put it better myself, except to add that there is no magic bullet or wand waving based solution.

Obesity is an example of a non-communicable disease, which means it cannot be spread by the same mechanisms by which infectious diseases are spread. The condition is for most of us an acquired characteristic meaning that if you are avoiding (or at least limiting) processed foods then you are unlikely to become obese. Having stated that, there is a large body of research which infers a genetic basis for obesity, which will not be discussed here. Suffice to say in this frame, the requirements of the body have been met but the hypothalamus does not respond to the action of hormones such as leptin and consequently the person takes longer to experience the sensation of feeling full. It is completely fair to state that there is a strong element of individual and community responsibility for obesity, but as the previous chapter sets out this is only part of the explanation. The simplest and most obvious mechanism by which to obviate the obesity epidemic is to shape food choices by ensuring that healthy eating options are affordable, accessible and readily available. In other words the elimination of food deserts and providing facilities by which people can exercise regularly and within their budget, all of this of course requires investment. Unfortunately, in the UK such funding is woefully lacking, for instance the FFLP partnership mentioned in Chapter 3 is almost totally dependent on funding from the national lottery, in my view this is akin to using a sticking plaster to treat a gangrenous wound. The FFLP is proven mechanism by which to improve the diet of millions of children and should be rolled nationally as a matter of priority. It is these sorts of initiatives that will enable the recommendations of agencies such as the MGI to translate into the necessary level of action. Intertwined with such a position is the role of the food industry and their bedfellows, the supermarkets. One could write an encyclopaedia on this relationship but one of its consequences is the fact that as of 2014 UK citizens are spending billions of pounds every year on ready meals. Some of his expenditure is in response to the on-going recession, whereby so called "*high end lines*" or "*supermarket take away boxes*" are substituting eating out. However, the fact remains that the UK ranks top of the ready meal consumption league, at least as far as Europe is concerned. Overall the UK has the worst obesity statistics in Europe, but only just. The bottom line is that the food industry must share the responsibility for the obesity problem alluded to in the previous chapters, to suggest otherwise is a cognitive dissonance bordering on denial. Put simply, the manufacturers should be compelled to move away from processed foods such as ready meals which are generally loaded with fat, sugar, salt and more individual additives and "*E*" numbers than there are characters on my key board. Furthermore there should be a massive program of diverting resources toward making healthy eating choices available at the expense of processed foods. The industry as a whole should be regulated such that, as one positive development, it is illegal to advertise junk food to children and teenagers. Such regulations ought to apply to the global junk food outlets. Again, this is not an exhaustive list it is only a scratch on the surface, but if obesity is to be genuinely treated as the new smoking then these are exactly the kind of initiatives which need to be pushed forward with the utmost urgency. According to the MGI report a reduction of obesity levels to 1993 levels will eliminate 5 million cases of obesity related disease and save the NHS at least £1 Billion annually. To put it alternatively the totality of interventions suggested in the MGI report could (according to its researchers) bring a fifth of obese and overweight people to a BMI which is less than 25. To my mind this is an absolute minimum. OK so there we have the big picture to coin the phrase "*what can you and I do, right now immediately, forthwith and with great gusto?*"

In my view the simplest way to integrate Sirtfoods into your diet is to go through the recipes in your favourite cook book. What's that you say, "*You don't have a cook book*", well, if you don't have a good cook book then you are in remiss, so you must get hold of one. I mean for sure there are thousands of recipes on line and dozens of exceptionally talented chefs with equally honed communication skills to help you cook them. That is all well and good, but a decent cookbook is absolutely essential for any kitchen. Speaking personally I am not a fan of what is called "*nouveau cuisine*" and I simply cannot abide restaurants that are all style and no substance. Think large plates with equally large prices but oppositely sized servings and you'll see where I am coming from. In short I see it as pretentious nonsense and equally the inverse of proper wholesome food. Ok that's that sorted! So what type of cook book should you get? Well there really is no set answer and you certainly don't need a brand new one. I got the two I use the most from a charity shop; others were picked up at the local car boot sale. Speaking personally I come from the no nonsense step by step explanation of how to make everything from a decent omelettes or full (variation in a theme) English breakfasts to gourmet meals that are designed to impress. Step forward roasted guinea fowl with pomegranate and braised greens (kale and spinach) with roasted vegetables, or for a 90% vegan like myself, all the above minus the Guinea Fowl.

My favourite style of cook book is the traditional farmhouse type or those of the Delia Smith variety. The reason is simple there are sections on how to make and prepare every dish you can conceivably think of. In fact such books are mine of information and contain all the advice you could possibly need plus the necessary nutritional advice as well as the definite no-no's. In this world of celebrity chefs I love the no-nonsense style of Nigel Slater and Gordon Ramsey (although the expletives are not always necessary, but hey that's marketing for you!). I have to say I have a healthy respect for Jamie Oliver, simply because the man can cook and constantly talks about "connecting with food", but more so for his tireless work to bring healthy foods to the schools and general public. A further piece to advice is to get your proverbial pantry filled with some staple ingredients that is herbs, spices, pulses, as well as various seasonings and flavourings. Many of which add to your SA's by default!

There is no great mystery to cooking, cheffing up, getting something together and most definitely quick and fast does not mean junk food. Put simply, if you can read a book and operate a cooker then you are able to eat healthily; even if some meals are somewhat unorthodox! For example consider the omelette my girlfriend has just made, a loose interpretation of a 30 year old Delia Smith recipe. Another reason why I love the more traditional and basic looking books, is to state that *"if it's not broken, it doesn't need fixing"*. The Sirtfood contingent is composed of olives and onions whilst the eggs bind together mushrooms tomatoes, one roast potato, a slice of stuffing, a smidgen of grated cheddar and some baked beans. All of it gently fried in a very thin layer of olive oil. Yes it's left over surprise, but it contains ALL the food groups and took 10 minutes to make. In addition, the moral aspects are satisfied, after all we live in a world were about 1Billion people are going without enough to eat, thus it is totally unacceptable to throw food away. So when you are cooking do not be stingy, but don't overdo it either and any excess should be portioned up for those times when you are in a hurry.

OK, back to the omelette! I am now fully energised and nutritionally stocked up until tea time when we will be having a Sirt food laden meal (courtesy of kale) tomato sauce with pasta. The great thing about making any sauce is that as long as you get the proportions about right you can make as much as you like. So you can make a shed load and then freeze what you don't use for another time. At this point it's worth pointing out that you could do with having some frozen stocks in your freezer. Believe me, freezing any surplus or intentionally making more than you need does save you time in the long run.

Chapter 6:
SIRT proteins, Activation and Processes Affected

"Today, more than 95% of all chronic disease is caused by food choice, toxic food ingredients, nutritional deficiencies and lack of physical exercise." Mike Adams (The Health Ranger and Natural News editor)

Metabolism is a complex series of inter-related biological processes which work collectively to maintain homoeostasis. In biology homoeostasis refers to maintaining every conceivable metabolic or biological process you can think of, irrespective of external conditions, within optimal conditions. For example your body temperature is not maintained at 37°C because it's a nice integer. The dissipation of the heat released as glucose is oxidised in the mitochondria and is regulated to maintain a body temperature of 37°C. This temperature is the optimum for the thousands of enzymes, including the SIRT enzymes which are so crucial to our metabolism. If this temperature is not maintained due to conditions such as hyperthermia (heat exhaustion), then many enzymes are said to denature. In one sentence this means that they lose the ability to catalyse metabolic reactions and so the processes that keep us alive begin to slow down or in extreme cases can actually stop altogether. Other variables such as acidity (pH levels) govern the efficiency of enzymes. For instance, salivary amylase will function in the near neutral (pH 6.2-7.4) conditions of the mouth. However, it would denature completely in the stomach where the protease enzymes are designed to work in the extremely acidic conditions of the stomach. An additional example concerns the role of anti-oxidants, and yes we are returning to this notion of a balanced diet. If too many anti-oxidants are consumed through feeding (or more likely they are ingested in supplement form), then the immune system can become compromised. Put simply the immune system requires minimum levels of free radicals (which will be discussed below), in the lymphatic and circulatory systems. In a related frame there is research from Scandinavia which asserts that excessive concentrations of anti-oxidants, actually promotes the growth of certain tumours, at least in laboratory animals. Furthermore, and perhaps to demonstrate the point that eating healthily beats supplements hands down other research indicates that too much resveratrol may nullify the proven benefits of regular exercise. These studies concerned excessively high doses of resveratrol which are far in excess of those one could expect from normal eating habits. This chapter will hopefully inculcate that compounds such as resveratrol are likely to have multiple roles in a properly functioning metabolism. Hence the reader is once again asked to sear that word balance and its slightly nerdy cousin homeostasis into their consciousness.

Resveratrol is thought to induce the production of a substance called endothelial nitric oxide, which stimulates the dilation of blood vessels. An endothelium is any layer of cells which covers any organ, but is most associated with vessels of the lymphatic and circulatory system. Hence resveratrol may have a role in maintaining an optimum body temperature during periods of exercise and exposure to high ambient temperatures. From this position research has indicated that resveratrol may play a part in alleviating hypertension. Other studies considered the role of supplements as opposed to consuming Sirtfoods properly. That is consumed as they were meant to be eaten, in leaf or berry form and not as dietary supplement pill. It has (I hope) been well established that diet is preferable to supplements and that field of SIRT protein research could lead to quantifiable benefits in terms of reducing obesity (malnutrition) in the industrialised world. We have established that eating Sirtfoods as part of a future and state run healthy eating programme would result in a massive reduction in obesity levels. However this statement does not explain the biochemical mechanisms which need to be functioning properly to achieve it. In other words it is self-evident that calorific restriction and ditching the junk and processed food will get your BMI down to the correct level, but how does this occur in biochemical terms?

Well first we need to explain what is meant by calorific restriction (CR), it's important because all of the processes outlined below are much more effective if the person is restricting their intake of unhealthy foods. OK here we go, CR as the term suggests is a mechanism by which it is possible to ingest all of your nutritional requirements without piling on the calories. In dietary terms a calorie is a unit employed to measure the energy content (as opposed to nutritional content) of a given food. All circumstances being equal the more calories that you ingest the more chance you have of becoming overweight or obese and/ or the more exercise you need to partake in. As we saw in the opening chapters the Sirtfoods are a range of high nutrient low energy foods. It must also be said that the more plant based matter that is eaten as compared with meat and to a lesser extent fish, the less calories you will ingest. In the context of obesity one does not need a PhD to assert that removing saturated fats will very quickly reduce your calorie intake. Research in the field of CR stretches back to the early years of the 20th century, but it is only in the last few years that mechanisms have been established which explain how it may work in the body. Overall, under the instruction of health professional CR will have benefits to a person provided it does not lead to malnutrition. In particular it has been shown to promote longevity and one mechanism by which this is thought to occur is through a process known as autophagy.

As stated in chapter one, living cells are the building blocks from which all organisms are made. As with all means of construction, the tools will eventually wear out and the same is true of cells and their components (the organelles). For instance red blood cells are manufactured in the bone marrow to replace those that are worn out and transported to the liver and spleen, where they are broken down. Every day approximately 2 million red blood cells are removed and replaced without compromising the ability of the blood stream to fulfil its transport function. The same is true of sub-cellular processes and the organelles which make them possible. In autophagy damaged or worn organelles are removed and replaced and the scientific literature imparts that SIRT1 has significance for the autophagy of mitochondria. From here it can be inferred that other SIRT proteins are involved in the autophagy of other organelles and that the homeostatic balance between removal of old organelles and the creation of new structures is an essential component of healthy metabolism. Such inferences have yet to be formally demonstrated but a role for the SIRT proteins is considered to be a possibility. However, a word of caution must be expressed to the reader.

Any assertion that a substance will increase the lifespan of any organism is sure to raise a few eyebrows and be greeted with a degree of popular and scientific scepticism. I mean let's be honest, the life extending properties of one substance or another have been extolled by different human cultures for thousands of years. It is well understood that in the ancient world the deities worshipped were seen as immortal by the mere puny mortals that worshipped them. In most of these cultures the source of immortality was normally connected to some form of food or infusion (elixir) that only the deity concerned was allowed to consume. A cursory look through the mythology of the ancient world makes reference to substances such as ambrosia or noma which could be consumed to extend the life of the mortals (that is people). Accordingly, the notion that SRT1 could extend the life of the common fruit fly (the Drosophila species so beloved of biological research) and certain nematodes, let alone human beings, has rightly been greeted with a healthy dose of solid scientific doubt. However, ever since the discovery in 2012 that SIRT6 could increase longevity in mice by 15%, interest in this aspect of sirtuin biology has far from waned. Evidence for longevity comes from a 2006 study which showed that mice that had been genetically engineered to be deficient in SIRT6 displayed the characteristics of ageing much more rapidly than their peers. The compound SIRT6 is believed to have a role in repairing cellular DNA and the transgenic mice that were lacking in this protein had all died within a month. When one considers that the life span of the average mouse is about a year, the implications are obvious. However, it cannot be stated that any of the sirtuin proteins is directly involved in prolonging the life of any mammalian species.

Additionally, the SIRT proteins do not operate in isolation from each other and as such they are likely to be involved in different biochemical processes. It is also not outside the bounds of possibility to state that the different modes of action are likely to have synergistic benefits to the organism. For instance in the above research the transgenic mice had been genetically engineered to develop malignant tumours. Concurrently, SIRT6 is widely believed to have a role in preventing certain cancers so if a mouse is deficient in that particular protein then the likelihood of developing tumours will increase. In other words there is no direct causative evidence that SIRT 6 or indeed the other Sirt promote longevity per se. What can be said with a high degree of confidence is that the Sirt proteins in general and SIRT6 in particular could affect the incidence of the biological characteristics of ageing. In addition, there is more than anecdotal evidence that the conditions associated with the ageing of the SIRT6 deficient mice could have been down to the consequences of excessively low and chronically depressed blood sugar levels. A further factor is gender. Irrespective of any research concerning Sirt proteins in mice, female mice live longer than male mice. In male mice that have been engineered to over express SIRT6 the animals simply caught up with the females who were the control or placebo group. In this frame it is important to remember that with homo-sapiens and many other mammals, there are good sound biological and evolutionary reasons as to why females live longer than males. Sorry guys (including yours truly) but the chances are that a far as longevity is concerned it will be a *"beast behind the door"* scenario, written by the internationally acclaimed author *"Hugo First"*.

In Secondary school one of the first metabolic processes that students learn about is aerobic respiration. Hence it seems appropriate to explore how calorific restriction and Sirtfoods could well benefit this most fundamental metabolic process. Glucose is the simplest carbohydrate and is the principle source of energy in living cells. The aerobic (oxygen present) respiration which occurs in every cell of our bodies is in effect a combustion reaction. In the mitochondria a complex series of reactions converts glucose to carbon dioxide and water and provide the energy needed for metabolism. Often the mitochondria are referred to as the power house of a healthy cell. For every mole (chemical counting unit) of glucose that is oxidised (reacted in the presence of oxygen) approximately 2830KJ (686 kilo calories) of energy is released. This works out to be approximately 4 calories per gram of glucose. In chemical reactions energy is obtained via the breaking of chemical bonds. The energy is not created it is transferred from the glucose molecules to an intermediary known as Adenosine Tri-Phosphate (ATP) which then transfers the energy through the cell. Often ATP will be referred to as the energy currency of living cells. There is a hefty amount of research which holds that SIRTSs 3-5 may finely tune the rate of respiration such that it occurs in line with the rate of nutrient (glucose) supply. In addition as ATP transfers chemical energy throughout the cell it is broken down, the only way it can be reused as the energy currency is if it is rebuilt back into ATP. This process is termed oxidative phosphorylation and is catalysed by SIRT 3. In addition SIRT 3 is thought to influence ketosis in the liver as well as the rate of ammonia removal during the breakdown of amino acids in the liver. Ketosis is the first stage of the fatty acid breakdown outlined below.

Further research in the activity of SIRT5 in this vital metabolic function continues apace. As stated above the SIRT proteins are likely to have a variety of functions and their activity can equally likely be triggered by different metabolic circumstances. For instance, if the body reduces its nutrient intake such that person is effectively fasting SIRT 1 protein has been shown to have a role in the function of the mitochondria in organs such as the liver and in the muscle fibres. The research literature is replete with indicators that the rate at which the cells construct mitochondria could be influenced by how energetic the cell is, that is the rate at which it is respiring. Overall, the supposition is that the presence of certain nutrients may act as a trigger to SIRT 1 (and to a lesser extent SIRT 3) and that in turn may increase the rate at which respiration occurs. In other words if you are following a Calorific Restriction / Sirtfood diet your cells are receiving more nutrients and glucose molecules and are functioning more efficiently. They are in effect operating within homeostatic limits. Metabolic diseases such as obesity are correlated with malfunctioning mitochondria. A further strand of research which may have implications for the treatment of diabetes is the presence (or not) of a hormone known as adiponectin, a protein and hormone that is only secreted from fat (adipose) cells. Adiponectin has a direct influence on the metabolism of fats and carbohydrates such as glucose. Its action has also been linked to the activity and presence of SIRT 1. Studies conducted on laboratory animals show that increasing levels of adiponectin in the general circulation provokes increased mitochondrial activity and by association the construction of mitochondria inside the cell. (Personally I do not support vivisection or any other type of animal experimentation but I feel I have to report the research and insights deduced). In addition because proteins are coded for by our DNA this relationship may well add extra weight to arguments concerning the genetic basis of obesity.

Related to the respiration of glucose is the metabolism of lipids (fats). In their entirety fats are an energy reserve which is stored as a layer of adipose (subcutaneous) tissue which is found on the lower end of the dermis (the skin) and has the dual function of acting as an insulating layer (fats are poor conductors of heat). A third function for fats in the body is to carry fat soluble vitamins to the cells of the body which use them. In other words fats are essential molecules, the trick is to modulate your intake and ingest the correct type that is the unsaturated variety. Fats are formed by two principle actions; first three soluble fatty acid molecules are chemically bonded to a substance known as glycerol. Hence fat molecules are often referred to as tri-glycerides. The second mechanism is through the action of insulin and that means we must very quickly revisit glucose. In the blood stream when glucose levels reach a high enough level the hypothalamus (part of the brain that controls homeostasis) sends a hormonal signal to the pancreas so that specialist cells known as "*beta*" cells secrete the hormone insulin. This stimulates all cells in the body to take up glucose and convert it to glycogen. This effect is most pronounced in the liver where the glycogen is stored until it is needed. The process that produces glycogen is known as glycolysis, thus glycogen is in effect thousands of individual glucose molecules attached to each other by what is termed a glycosidic bond. Hence, both glucose and glycogen are readily available energy sources whose relative concentrations are regulated by the action of the hormones insulin and glucagon. The latter hormone is released when glucose levels fall low enough for the hypothalamus to signal the "*alpha*" cells in the pancreas to release it. The release of glucagon stimulates the liver to convert the glycogen back into glucose (glucogenesis) by breaking the glycosidic bonds between each glucose molecule in the glycogen molecule. This another example of homeostasis and when the system breaks down type 2 diabetes can develop (Type 1 is ignored for the purpose of this writing). It is well established that Sirts-3-5 congregate around the mitochondria. Thus, it is fair to assert that Sirts3-5 are likely to have an essential role in regulating cellular respiration.

Once all cells in the body have enough glucose to meet their needs and the liver and muscles are packed with glycogen, glucose is converted to fatty acid and in turn chemically bonded to the glycerol molecule and then transported to the adipose layer. If a person is overweight or obese they do not necessarily have more fat cells than a person who is not. It is more that each fat cell contains more fat molecules. Once you have accumulated excess fat it is very difficult to remove unless you change your diet, principally, because fats are such a concentrated store of energy. It takes a lot of exercise before the body starts to break down fatty acids in aerobic respiration. Hence, the best course of action is prevention as opposed to cure! In very general terms the body will use its reserves of glucose and glycogen before it starts to break down fat reserves. A diet rich in Sirtfoods and plant matter in general contains more nutrients and fewer carbohydrates than the western diet outlined previously. Hence you are less likely to gain weight via the ingestion of nutritionally questionable foods. In extreme cases of obesity that may require surgery to remove excess fat a surgeon or doctor will likely prescribe a calorific restriction diet regime. This is simply because the body has to start burning off its stores of fat and won't do that whilst the person is still ingesting carbohydrates. Fats are much more concentrated store (as opposed to source) of energy. On average each mole of fat contains approximately 9 grams of energy and we have between 50 and 200 billion fat cells. Once your sugar levels are being properly maintained the body can start breaking down the fatty acids. SIRT3 is thought to have a function in the oxidation of fatty acids, which is the first stage of their breakdown. The trick is to get your body into a position to start the metabolism of fat cells. The first stage of which is the ketosis mentioned above.

If you are overweight or obese the only way you are going to burn off your excess fat is by avoiding foods which are high in refined sugar and fats. That is foods which are the total opposite of Sirtfoods and its more proscriptive variant the calorific restriction (C.R.) diet. Your body will use glucose and glycogen first and if you keep ingesting excessive carbohydrates (which are metabolised to sugars such as glucose) all you will succeed in doing is replenishing your reserves of glucose or worse actually increasing your BMI. You will need to follow a genuinely balanced diet in which fresh Sirtfoods will play a part. Or follow the instructions of a surgeon pertaining to a CR diet. Helpfully, SIRT1 and SIRT3 have been shown to have a function in detecting the presence of the products of digestion. These products are in effect the nutrients the body needs and their presence (or not) influences the activity of other proteins inside the mitochondria. Perhaps to underline the point about balance, in instances of caloric restriction (i.e. fasting), SIRT 3 in effect goes into overdrive. The protein will activate and then inhibit the action of a whole range of enzymes and protein function in general and in this context SIRT 3 has been associated with modulating conditions ranging from the cardiovascular to diabetes and hearing loss.

SIRT1 is found in many mammals and is most active when feeding is problematic for the organism. It is equally active when a calorific restriction (CR) diet is imposed. It also has a fundamental role in the biology of free radical clean-up which is discussed below. It is also considered to have a profound role in regulating the cell cycle and therefore cellular lifespan. This assertion clearly has implications for the treatment of cancer and stress related conditions. As a regulator of metabolism and respiration it is known to accelerate the rate at which cells aerobically convert glucose to its metabolites (CO_2 and H_2O). Furthermore SIRT1 has been shown to suppress the storage of fats whilst simultaneously increasing the rate of processes such as ketosis. Thus SIRT1 can potentially reduce the incidence of conditions ranging from heart attacks to osteoporosis, in short the conditions associated with both obesity and old age. It must be restated that science is a long way from demonstrating the exact mechanisms by which all the SIRT compounds garner their metabolic benefits, but the research is continuing. Overall good diet raises the levels of SIRT 1 and there is no reason to suppose that the same effect can be produced with the other 6 SIRT compounds.

Any discussion of SIRT proteins would be incomplete without some mention of substances known as free radicals. In what is perhaps one of the great ironies of life on planet Earth, the production of certain types (species) of charged atoms of oxygen are known to have a damaging effect on the biological molecules which are essential for cell integrity and function. Other species of atom such as hydrogen and nitrogen are also known to exert similar effects which fall under the term *"Cellular Oxidative Stress"* (COS). It is molecules referred to as free radicals that are thought to promote COS, so we must ask how this works. Electrons are the sub-atomic and negatively charged particles which occupy the empty space around the nucleus. When an atom is electrochemically balanced the number of positively charged protons (in the nucleus) will equal the number of electrons which spin around the nucleus in electron clouds. Electrons themselves are most stable when they exist together in pairs. A free radical forms in atoms when the electron pairs are split and the particles are separated from each other. Such separation of electron pairs is a common feature of many biological processes. A free radical is a highly energetic form of an atomic substance and for our purposes we are most interested in oxygen. In a free radical state the species of atom is seeking to off load its surplus of energy and in the firing line are biological molecules ranging from fats to Deoxy-Ribonucleic Acid (DNA). The phrase *"COS"* is a catch all term used to describe damage caused by reactive oxygen species (ROS). In other words any molecule which carries at least one unpaired electron can cause damage to biological molecules inside living cells as well as those which exist on its membrane. However, there is no need to panic! It all comes back to the phrase *"balanced diet"*. Provided the diet contains an abundance of anti-oxidants, the impact of the free radicals is curtailed.

In their entirety the SIRT enzymes are widely believed to protect cells from the attentions of free radical molecules which love nothing better than to pass on their excess energy to any takers. They in effect promote the activity of other biological molecules (not limited to enzymes), such that excess free radicals are chemically reduced. You may recall from secondary (high) school chemistry the mnemonic (OILRIG). The initials refer to the movement of electrons and they mean oxidation is loss and reduction is gain of electrons. In chemistry the reactivity of a substance is determined by the position and numbers of electrons which are furthest from the nucleus. Atomic theory shows us that the negatively charged electrons orbit the nucleus in orbital clouds and they are held in place by the protons of the nucleus, which have a positive charge. An atom is said to be electrochemically stable when the number of electrons and protons is equal. The electrons themselves are most stable when they orbit the nucleus in pairs. During the course of our metabolism it is perfectly normal for radical species such as reactive oxygen species (ROS) to be produced. Hence we have over millions of years evolved processes which effectively hoover up the free radicals which *"can"* (emphasis) cause damage to biological molecules in, on and around the cell. These species of atom are reactive because they have so much excess energy; the only way they can lose this energy is by chemically reacting with any substance that they come into contact with. When this happens the free radical is chemically reduced and the biological molecule is oxidised. Hence for chemical reactions which involve reduction and oxidation the term *"redox"* is applied and both processes occur simultaneously.

The compound which is oxidised loses its electrons to the substance it is reacting with; hence the second reacting substance is reduced. Now, to really confuse you! A substance which is termed a *"reducing agent"* is said to cause oxidation because the reducing agent causes the oxidised substance to lose electrons to the reducing agent. In other words the oxidised substance loses electrons and the reduced substance gains the *same* electrons. Conversely an "oxidising agent" is said to cause reduction because it loses electrons to a second reacting substance, which is itself reduced. Practically all chemical reactions fall under the term *"redox"* and if you're flummoxed don't worry. Please feel free to read this section again and follow up on the previous hyperlinks! For our purposes all you need to appreciate is that the free radical is the reducing agent and the biological molecules are the source of extra electrons. The Sirt proteins are believed to act themselves as either the electron source or more likely activate so called oxygen scavenging substances. For example SIRT 3 has been shown to activate enzymes which are prolific scavengers of reactive oxygen species (ROS). In other words the anti-oxidant reduces the free radicals it comes into contact while it is simultaneously oxidised. In so doing the free radical loses electrochemical energy to the anti-oxidant and not to essential biological molecules. This underpins a fundamental tenet of chemical reactivity. Namely, that substances react with each other to become more energetically stable and that as this stability is achieved, no new electrons are made, they are transferred or shared between reacting substances, forming new compounds in the process. Overall, the SIRT proteins appear to have definite function in regulating COS

"*Cellular Oxidative Stress*" and so may have an indirect effect in curtailing the development of degenerative disease and other less serious conditions that are associated with aging.

Stress is a highly subjective occurrence and is expressed differently in different people, irrespective of the circumstances. In biological terms stress occurs when the body responds in a physiological manner due to the result of a stimulus or sensory input. The stress response is highly beneficial to the survival of the organism; one must only look at the "*fight or flight*" response to see this assertion exemplified. In its entirety stress is an entirely predictable and normal biological occurrence which induces a change in behaviour which is designed to remove the organism from the stressing event or enable it to be accommodated. The physiological basis of the stress response is the action of the hormones Cortisol and noradrenalin which are secreted from the adrenal glands situated on the kidneys. The stress response signals the body that it has to prepare by either "*fighting*" or "*flighting*" or possibly both and is only beneficial while the event is occurring. A huge burst of energy fuelled by the aerobic respiration of glucose promotes the feeling of being alert and primed for action. This is a normal facet of our evolution and is absolutely essential to our survival. Consider what would happen if you did not respond quickly and rapidly to a fast moving vehicle that was coming right at you? The same question could be asked of the first humans as they sought to avoid predation.

Problems begin to develop when the feeling of being "*stressed*" is regular and / or constant. Consequently, the body does not have the opportunity to re-adjust back to a less stressed state. Stress hormone levels can reach very high levels in the blood stream which can present serious health risks not dissimilar to those associated with obesity. In other words chronic stress results in systemic changes to the biochemistry and metabolism of the stressed person. These changes announce their impact in the form of diseases or conditions including:

- Circulatory and pulmonary systems (heart, lungs and circulation)

- Obesity and related conditions such as diabetes

- Hypertension

- Immune system where the functioning of B and T cells is impaired

- Insomnia and associated depression and lethargy

- Osteoporosis and other physical conditions associated with ageing

- Dementia including but not limited to Alzheimer's disease

In terms of neurological impacts elevated and chronic levels of cortisol in the blood stream are viewed as dangerous because of the impact on the hippocampus (part of the brain which deals with memory and thought). Although no causative link has as yet been established the evidence suggests that the brains of highly stressed persons are smaller than those of their unstressed counterparts. The culprit being a reduced volume hippocampus which is implicated in the memory and cognitive deficits associated with dementia. It is important to underline that the stress response itself is not dangerous; however, being in a heightened state of stress as result of a messy divorce, a workplace dispute or even the bi-daily rush hour can all trigger a long term stress response. The list of triggers is endless and will almost certainly be different for different people. To avoid the risks associated with elevated levels of stress hormones the body needs time to break them down into harmless substances which can either be re-assimilated or expelled. In what is known as the cortisol / adrenal switch the time taken for cortisol and nor-adrenaline to become toxins is limited. In other words the time taken for a substance to start behaving as a toxin has a major influence on how the body deals stressing events. If the body does not have time to cope with stressing events then the beneficial aspects of the stress response are morphed into a set of symptoms (such as those mentioned above) which can be catastrophic for the person.

In all human cells (aside from the gametes and red blood cells) there are 23 pairs of chromosomes. These are the structures which contain the molecules of DNA and on the end of each DNA molecule is a structure known as a telomere. The complete structure and function of telomeres is not fully understood but they have a vital role in keeping living cells biologically fit for purpose. With each cell division the telomeres become shorter and hence cells have a limited lifespan. One facet of the biology of a chronically stressed person is the extent to which their stress is expressed at a cellular level. The disappearance of telomeres causes a condition known as cellular senescence, where the cell is alive but no longer capable of reproduction. This process is widely believed to be the genetic basis for ageing. In people who are chronically stressed the action of the hormone cortisol interferes with the enzyme telomerase which catalysis the chemical reactions that repair telomeres. As an example of why the diet must be balanced it is recognised that excessive amounts of ECGC inhibit the action of telomerase and the processes which manufacture proteins in the ribosome's.

In certain species of yeast SIRT2 has been observed to help prolong the life of individual cells. Research shows us that SIRT2 is most present in the cell during asexual reproduction (mitosis) where they congregate around the chromosomes as they divide. To be precise the SIRT 2 proteins congregate around a single strand of DNA (a chromatid) which is found in the nucleus of the daughter cell immediately after it has separated from the parent cell. Clearly, this suggests a role for this protein in the successful reproduction of living cells. Thus if ageing is directly associated with reduction in the length of telomeres and if SIRT2 is associated with dividing chromosomes and therefore the successful copying of genetic information, then a confluence of stress, SIRT activity and diet clearly presents itself. SIRT1 is widely believed to contribute to the free radical clean up outlined in the section on free radicals. Any substance which reduces the impact of *"Cellular Oxidative Stress"* must by definition contribute to the over health of the person (or other living organism). SIRT1 has been shown to catalyse the biochemical reactions which hoover up the free radical substances in the manner described above. In addition SIRT1 has been shown to have a role in maintaining an optimal telomere length and because it is known to contribute to what geneticists call gene silencing it could influence the onset of age related diseases that have a genetic basis. This is a convenient juncture at which to point out that when we are referring to the longevity benefits of Sirtuin Activators (SA's) we are talking about treating conditions associated with ageing. If this conditions can be treated such as through stem cell science then they may well contribute to a longer life span. You are still going to "age" in the truest sense of the word but it is entirely possible that the biological conditions we associate with old age may well become treatable.

At the same time SIRT2 may well have a role in ensuring that the enzymes which are responsible for copying DNA and synthesising new proteins function properly. Overall SIRT2 may have a role in regulating the success and rate of protein synthesis and the recombination of DNA during mitosis as well as ensuring that the sub-telomeric region of each DNA molecule is properly maintained. This is the region of each chromosome just next to each telomere and is thought to act as a buffer between the telomere and the rest of the DNA strand. However, the exact mechanism(s) by which all of these processes occur are far from being understood. It can be stated that stress and stress management are strongly connected to the biochemistry of the active substances bound up in the Sirtfoods. Additionally, chronic stress induces a situation where metabolism is well out of balance, or homeostatically challenged if you wish to be technical! Hence, if eating well can form part of an overall stress elimination (or at least management) program then consuming Sirtfoods may contribute to alleviating the genetic basis for ageing and could act as an insurance policy in terms of the health of the cell. Furthermore, cortisol_and other hormones are known to suppress the immune system and so stress, telomeres and Sirtfoods could collectively have a role in maintaining defence against pathogens. The question is how we as individuals mediate between a normal and healthy stress response and a chronic, constant and consistent stress response. Intertwined with this question is the role of consuming a Sirt food rich diet in keeping stress levels down and the immune system functioning. Hence a further strand of Sirt food consumption is to reduce such symptoms but diet alone is not going to provide a person with the space they need to deal with their stress. I mean let us be clear all the healthy eating in the world is not in itself going to fix the stresses caused by a consistently punishing work schedule or fix the relationship problems which are known to be caused by a work life balance that is skewed in the wrong direction, (i.e. toward work in case you were wondering).

Chapter 7:
A Concise History of Sirtfood Research

"Man Is What He Eats" Titus Lucretius Carus (99 BC – 55 BC) was a Roman poet and philosopher

The year 2008 is a convenient start date for providing a context for research into the biochemistry of Sirtuin foods and Sirtuin Activators. In this year GlaxoSmithKline (GSK) for the tidy sum of $720 million brought out a US biotechnology firm called Sirtris Pharmaceuticals. The company was founded in 2004 by a Harvard biology graduate named Brian Sinclair. The interest of GSK was piqued because Sirtrus Pharmaceuticals were researching the role of compounds such as resveratrol and other polyphenol compounds in SIRT protein activation. It is the polyphenols which are recognised to contribute to the free radical clean up outlined below. In particular GSK were interested in the efficacy of a compound they named SRT-501, which contains resveratrol as its active ingredient. This of course begs an obvious question, *"what is resveratrol?"*

The precise chemical name for resveratrol is 3,5,4'-trihydroxystilbene which is manufactured by many autotrophs (plants) as a normal part of their metabolism. For instance the aggressively invasive Japanese knotweed synthesis this polyphenolic compound as a fungicide, which protects its roots from attack. In terms of our diet resveratrol is found in the skin of red grapes and so is helpfully found in copious amounts in all forms of red wine. Hurrah! It is also found in peanuts, dark chocolate and blue berries. Helpfully, all of these foods contain many of the vitamins (A through to K) and trace minerals (such as Iron and potassium), thus the healthy living benefits are self-evident and the potential efficacy of resveratrol an equally important bonus. In essence you can feel better about having peanut butter on toast, munching on your favourite peanuts during the football as well as grating dark chocolate on your blue berry and bananas in your morning muesli. While you're at it you can feel free to wash it all down with a wholly desirable glass of Rioja, maybe not with breakfast though. This is wonderfully convenient because it is the skin of fruits such as red grapes and berries are considered to be the most concentrated source of resveratrol.

The compound SRT 501 was of interest to GlaxoSmithKline because it is believed to have a role in activating the SIRT1 protein. One area of interest was in the in the treatment of multiple myeloma. This type of cancer arises from the blood plasma, which is the alkaline liquid through which nutrients and waste products are exchanged in the blood stream. Myeloma affects the white blood cells manufactured in the bone marrow (where red blood cells are also continually manufactured). Hence myeloma can affect the overall composition and therefore effectiveness of the blood as a transport medium. Myeloma has particular affinity for the white plasma cells involved in the production of anti-bodies, which are the proteins found on the cells of immune system. Antibodies function by recognising the antigens of pathogenic bacteria as well as virus particles and then the immune system is stimulated to destroy them. In the case of virus particles (such as those which cause the common cold) the body must manufacture sufficient quantities of the antibody carrying cells before the immune system is itself overwhelmed. Also known as immunoglobulins these antibodies are produced by white plasma cells on instruction from the T and B-cells of the immune system. Hence the plasma cells are crucial for a robust immune response and because these cells are manufactured in many bone marrow sites, myeloma can rapidly spread, hence the prefix "multiple". A person suffering from multiple myeloma has a severely degraded immune system. Thus, biological agents which would normally be harmless (or dealt with very quickly) can present a real danger to the health of the person. In effect the genetic make-up of the cells is changed such that they only manufacture a single anti-body called para-protein which has no known beneficial function. The presence of para protein is used to test for the presence of multiple myeloma. In many ways researching resveratrol is an example of a journey into the dark heart of the human condition.

Science is a human enterprise and despite it being one of the greatest achievements of our species scientists are not infallible and the literature is replete with instances of temptation and plain old scientific fraud fuelled by corruption. For example consider the U.S surgeon Dipak Das who in 2012 was found to have falsified data in 145 separate instances. Consequently said data was retracted including extensive work on the role of resveratrol in the treatment of heart disease. A further factor is the metabolism of resveratrol itself, the compound easily passes from the intestines to the liver. However, only about 1% of any ingested amount actually makes it to the blood stream. The compound is rapidly broken down and may well be converted to other substances before it can be transported to sites where it may express its potential benefits. Such poor bio-availability contrasts markedly with the action of resveratrol in vitro (outside the body) where it is applied to populations of micro-organisms in concentrations that have yet to be achieved in any clinical trial. At time of writing the only way to obtain to obtain these kinds of dose levels is in the form of supplements.

The promotion of these supplements almost exclusively focuses on their purported cosmetic benefits. Such marketing has absolutely nothing to do with the transport and metabolism of resveratrol and everything to do with exploiting insecurity. Without doubt these spurious claims ought to be categorically rejected. It is then unsurprising that research concerning the efficacy of synthetic derivatives of resveratrol continues apace. The question as to whether such derivatives should form part of a normal balanced diet will doubtless continue to present itself. As the reader can infer I am not a fan of certain supplements, however, it is not for me to preach, it is for the reader to make an informed choice. No matter your opinion, no supplement should be consumed without the knowledge or consent of your doctor. All of these indicators pertaining to the efficacy of resveratrol in human beings can be broken down into two basic suppositions. Either resveratrol is so potent that even tiny amounts garner physiological effects or that these effects are down to other metabolic factors that we have yet to determine. Concurrently, whether resveratrol and the other polyphenols have a role in chemo-prevention is a long way from being established.

In 2010 GlaxoSmithKline (GSK) ceased all clinical trials which used SRT-501 as an agent to counter the effects of multiple myeloma. In short it just didn't work and caused wholly undesirable side effects ranging from renal (kidney) failure to vomiting and diarrhoea, which then lead to dehydration. Clearly, just what you need when you are suffering with cancer. Subsequently, it has been shown that resveratrol is not shy when it comes to bonding to receptors and the active sites of many enzymes. Meaning it can have a direct impacts on biochemical processes which may not benefit the person who has ingested too much of the chemical. In 2013 GSK shut down the subsidiary that it paid so much to acquire. This does not mean that research into Sirtuin Activators is dead and buried, quite the opposite, the potential is huge. As of 2015

GSK is continuing to research the efficacy of other plant based drugs. On top of all of this it must be remembered that we are talking about diet and not supplements. Many of the unpleasant side effects and other negative impacts which have occurred have been because the concentrations ingested have been so high. In other words the active ingredient has behaved as a toxin which the body will seek to remove by any means at its disposal. Research is now focusing on the metabolic pathways in which the chemicals in side Sirtfoods are thought to function. A key focus of the science is to find molecules which are much more selective than resveratrol and do not provoke side effects. In terms of chemo-prevention no such molecule that specifically targets the Sirtuin Activators (SA's) has been discovered. Red wine contains anything up to 14mg of resveratrol per litre and you must feel free to enjoy a glass of your favourite brew of alcoholic grape juice. Just don't expect it to be a panacea cure for undesirable biological conditions.

So what is the future of research into Sirt proteins and their activating chemicals? Well put simply it's bright and like all good science it's self-regulating and it learns from its mistakes. In this frame Sirtfood research ought to be viewed as an example of science operating at its best. The reader must appreciate that much of the literature published and science being conducted is occurring at the limits of our knowledge in this area. The next big discovery in the field could quite literally be around the next corner. The SIRT proteins are known to be most active when the body is metabolising within its optimal limits (homeostasis). This fact should imply that cellular health will be maintained and diseases such as cancer, diabetes and all the other conditions associated with western diet are nullified. Much of the current research and likely future research on Sirt proteins and their activators is concerned with using diet as a preventative measure to assuage these negative biological conditions. For instance a compound known as SIRT2104, (which seems to activate SIRT1) is undergoing what are termed *"initial safety studies"*. This is scientific parlance for the safety trials that are carried on volunteers who in this case are prone to type 2 diabetes and inflammatory diseases. The same compound has been postulated to have a role in treating aspects of crohn's disease and its equally unpleasant bed fellow IBS (Irritable Bowl Syndrome). However, please don't hold your breath; there is still a long way to go. Which gives us a helpful moment to reiterate that where ever possible prevention is better than cure?

Fundamentally there are 7 inter-related strands of research pertaining to the biochemistry andactivation of the SIRT proteins. One recent development concerns research published in 2014 which focuses on the SIRT6. It is known that the SIRT6 enzyme inhibits tumor growth in the liver and colon of laboratory animals. However, the same protein has been observed to promote the growth of skin cancer cells because it has been shown to activate the enzymes which induce skin tumor growth. In other words there is a possibility that exposure to UV-B radiation could negate the action of SIRT6, at least as far as the skin is concerned. The SIRT 6 enzyme does have an implicit role in protecting DNA from genomic instability but this research appears to indicate that this efficacy varies between tissue types and can be disrupted by external factors. The point here is that if you are going to catch some rays, you had better do it with moderation and especially be careful not to burn. The same research demonstrated that when laboratory mice were genetically engineered to not express SIRT6 the incidence of skin cancer was significantly reduced. The mode of action in this context concerns the relationship between SIRT6 and an enzyme known as COX-2. This enzyme is responsible for skin inflammation, cellular reproduction (mitosis) and it is known to extend the life span of skin cells. These processes are inextricably bound up in the proliferation of cancer cells. In this particular set of experiments when SIRT6 levels were increased so did skin cancer, when SIRT 6 levels were reduced so did the incidence of the cancer cells. In other words there is a direct correlation between the two variables. The research supposes that exposure to UV-B light promotes the activity of SIRT6 in skin cells and that this activity increase the production of the COX-2 enzyme. Overall, this single piece of research underpins the complexity of the science involved in SIRT protein science. On the one hand we know more about the onset of skin cancer, on the other science needs to establish ways to inhibit this expression without disrupting its other functions in the body.

Chapter 8:
A Final Word

"Let thy food be thy medicine and thy medicine be thy food" Hippocrates (460-377B.C.)

Some form of regular exercise is essential to achieving any degree of weight loss; now this does not have to mean joining a gym or pumping iron every day. It means riding your push bike or walking to work and leaving the car at home whenever you can. Clearly, you should consult your doctor or health practitioner for advice but I can guarantee that he or she will ask you about your eating habits. Your job is to take heed and follow as best you can their instructions. The trick is to maintain a healthy balance between eating, metabolism and exercise. Irrespective of an individual context the fact remains, if excess fat is allowed to accumulate then the person is sure to become *"overweight"* if things slip further the person may become a contributor to the *"global obesity epidemic"* alluded to elsewhere in this text. The more you exercise or the more active you are, the more carbohydrates and fats are "burned off" in the mitochondria. The reader should not be left with the impression that one particular aspect of their diet will definitely prevent the onset of cancer or indeed any other negative biological occurrence. In other words do not rush out and buy bags of green tea and expect not to develop cancer if you are not implementing other positive changes to your life style. Having stated that, the potential benefits of eating Sirtfoods as part of your normal healthy eating routine in this book cannot be understated. The substances thought to activate the SIRT proteins are, at their simplest, chemicals derived from the food that we eat. We obtain these chemicals through digestion and they are then used in their entirety to drive our metabolism. In other words all those lovely colours that you see in all the food you have ever eaten no matter the forms in which you ingest are made of chemicals. The chemicals which keep us alive are atoms of carbon, hydrogen, nitrogen, oxygen, phosphorous and sulphur which are arranged and chemically bonded together to form the compounds we eat. We also consume vitamins and minerals which are by and large made of the same atoms as well as fibre and water. In other words every substance that we eat and then digest has some sort of metabolic function. Of course it's self-evident that they will influence the biochemistry of the SIRT proteins and will be enhanced if they are regularly stocked up with the molecules we need to ingest irrespective of our knowledge of their existence. To me, that says Job done!

This book is the culmination of a long and sometimes painful journey from health to fitness. I had to completely re-evaluate what I thought I knew about food and even our society and the way it functions (that's for another book). It can be very challenging to face off old beliefs that are engrained from an early age about food. During this journey one of the most startling discoveries I made was that your regular MD has very little knowledge about diet and health. They seem to know the basics like everyone does but they never have time to specialise. It's much easier to treat a symptom with pharmaceuticals than to really understand and prevent the cause of the illness. I'm not looking for a bandage or a pill from my doctor; I want knowledge that prevents illness in the first place. Good health and ill health can be promoted by your own body; it just needs the correct fuel in the form of nutrition. If you eat dead food that's overly processed and full of additives and chemicals you will slowly starve your cells of nutrition and then the worst nightmares can and often will happen. The old hippy adage comes to mind "treat your body like a temple" or in today's zeitgeist "treat your body like a sports car". Make sure you have only the best quality fuel/food working in your body, your body deserves it. During our brief time here our bodies have a lot of work to do so treat it well. J. Hodges

Glossary of terms

Alveoli - any of the many tiny air sacs of the lungs which allow for rapid gaseous exchange.

Autophagy - is a normal physiological process in the body that deals with destruction of cells in the body. It maintains homeostasis or normal functioning by protein degradation and turnover of the destroyed cell organelles for new cell formation.

Carbonic Anhydrase - The **carbonic anhydrases** (or carbonate dehydratases) form a family of enzymes that **catalyze** the rapid interconversion of **carbon** dioxide and water to bicarbonate and protons (or vice versa), a reversible reaction that occurs relatively slowly in the absence of a catalyst.

CJD - **Creutzfeldt-Jakob disease** (CJD) is a rare, degenerative, invariably fatal brain disorder. [1] Although the agent of sporadic **CJD** (sCJD), the most common type of **CJD**, differs from the agent of bovine spongiform encephalopathy (BSE) or "mad cow disease", sCJD is often confused with the human form of BSE.

Cytoplasm - the material or protoplasm within a living cell, excluding the nucleus.

Cytosol - the aqueous component of the cytoplasm of a cell, within which various organelles and particles are suspended.

Enzymes - a substance produced by a living organism which acts as a catalyst to bring about a specific biochemical reaction.

Golgi - an organelle in eukaryotic cells that stores and modifies proteins for specific functions and prepares them for transport to other parts of the cell. The **Golgi** apparatus is usually near the cell nucleus and consists of a stack of flattened sacs

Homeostasis - the tendency towards a relatively stable equilibrium between interdependent elements, especially as maintained by physiological processes.

Homeostatically - The tendency of the body to seek and maintain a condition of balance or equilibrium within its internal environment, even when faced with external changes. A simple example of homeostasis is the body's ability to maintain an internal temperature around 98.6 degrees Fahrenheit, whatever the temperature outside.

Metabolites - a substance formed in or necessary for metabolism.

Mitosis - a type of cell division that results in two daughter cells each having the same number and kind of chromosomes as the parent nucleus, typical of ordinary tissue growth.

Organelles - any of a number of organized or specialized structures within a living cell.

Polyphenol - a compound containing more than one phenolic hydroxyl group.

Ribosomes - a minute particle consisting of RNA and associated proteins found in large numbers in the cytoplasm of living cells. They bind messenger RNA and transfer RNA to synthesize polypeptides and proteins.

U.N.E.S.C.O. - United Nations Educational, Scientific, and Cultural Organization.

W.H.O. – World Health Organisation

Useful Websites

http://nutritionfacts.org

http://www.naturalnews.com

http://nutritiondata.self.com

https://www.pinterest.com/coco942001/save-yourself/

https://www.pinterest.com/coco942001/clean-food-recipes/

https://viddapublishing.com

http://viddapublishing.blogspot.co.uk/

Sources

http://www.sciencedirect.com/science/article/pii/S0006295211005697

http://www.nejm.org/doi/full/10.1056/NEJMoa1200303

http://www.theguardian.com/science/blog/2014/apr/11/resveratrol-wonder-chemical-red-wine-cancer-ageing

http://www.xconomy.com/boston/2013/03/12/glaxosmithkline-shuts-down-sirtris-five-years-after-720m-buyout/

http://www.nature.com/neuro/journal/v1/n1/pdf/nn0598_69.pdf

http://www.theguardian.com/society/2014/nov/20/obesity-bigger-cost-than-war-and-terror

http://www.cancer.gov/about-cancer/causes-prevention/risk/diet/tea-fact-sheet

http://www.mdpi.com/1420-3049/12/5/946

http://www.nature.com/news/sirtuin-protein-linked-to-longevity-in-mammals-1.10074

http://ajcn.nutrition.org/content/81/2/341.full.pdf+html

http://www.rsc.org/chemistryworld/2013/06/resveratrol-red-wine-heart-disease-podcast

http://mcb.asm.org/content/23/9/3173.full.pdf+html

http://jnci.oxfordjournals.org/content/89/24/1881.full.pdf+html

http://cshperspectives.cshlp.org/content/4/12/a013102.full.pdf+html

http://www.sciencedirect.com/science/article/pii/S0925443913001804

http://www.sciencedirect.com/science/article/pii/S0009898112005773

http://sciencelife.uchospitals.edu/2014/10/16/two-faced-gene-sirt6-prevents-some-cancers-but-promotes-sun-induced-skin-cancer/

http://www.the-scientist.com/?articles.view/articleNo/13625/title/Mapping-Subtelomeres/

http://www.ncbi.nlm.nih.gov/pubmed/18607383

http://www.kurzweilai.net/why-sirt1-in-your-brain-may-keep-you-smart

http://www.ncbi.nlm.nih.gov/pmc/articles/PMC3249911/

http://www.ncbi.nlm.nih.gov/pmc/articles/PMC2727669/

http://www.ncbi.nlm.nih.gov/pmc/articles/PMC3117983/

http://www.chem.ucla.edu/harding/ec_tutorials/tutorial43.pdf

http://www.ncbi.nlm.nih.gov/pmc/articles/PMC2835915/

http://www.nature.com/ncomms/2014/140401/ncomms4557/full/ncomms4557.html

http://www.ncbi.nlm.nih.gov/pmc/articles/PMC2020845/#R10

http://www.ncbi.nlm.nih.gov/pmc/articles/PMC2020845/

http://www.sciencedaily.com/releases/2013/03/130327133341.html

http://www.theatlantic.com/health/archive/2014/03/science-compared-every-diet-and-the-winner-is-real-food/284595/

http://www.theguardian.com/lifeandstyle/2013/jun/19/japanese-diet-live-to-100

https://elainehastings.wordpress.com/tag/mediterranean-diet/

http://www.hindawi.com/journals/omcl/2013/707421/

http://genesdev.cshlp.org/content/27/19/2072.full.pdf+html

http://www.nature.com/cddis/journal/v1/n1/pdf/cddis200917a.pdf

http://www.nature.com/cddis/journal/v1/n1/pdf/cddis20098a.pdf

http://jn.nutrition.org/content/10/1/63.short

Books and further reading

Not on the label Felicity Lawrence, Penguin books 2004.

http://www.mckinsey.com/insights/economic_studies/how_the_world_could_better_fight_obesity

http://www.foodforlife.org.uk/what-is-food-for-life

http://www.nationalobesityforum.org.uk/media/PDFs/StateOfTheNationsWaistlineObesityintheUKAnalysisandExpectations.pdf

http://www.sciencedaily.com/search/?keyword=sirtuins+%2Bcalorie+restriction#gsc.tab=0&gsc.q=sirtuins%20%2Bcalorie%20restriction&gsc.page=1

Before you go

Thank you for purchasing my book!

If you found this book interesting and enjoyed reading it, I would really appreciate a short **review on Amazon**. All of your feedback is valuable to me, as your comments and input will be taken on board to help me make this and future books even better.

I would love hearing what you have to say. Please leave me a helpful REVIEW on Amazon.

Other Books by VIDDA Publishing

THE MEDICINE ON YOUR PLATE Series

Understanding Disease, Prevention & The Importance of Plant Based Nutrition and Diet

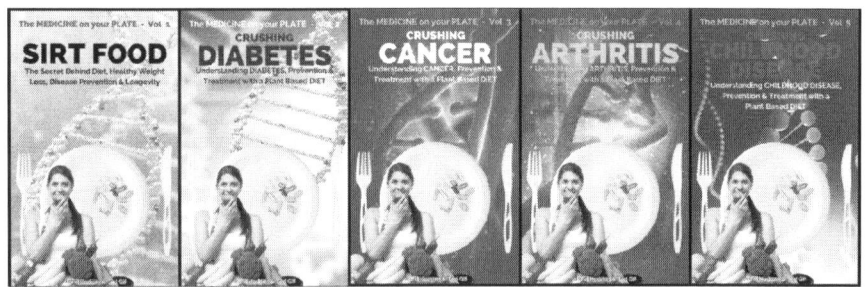

GREEN UP YOUR LIFE Series (Available in Spanish)
Take control of your health and wellbeing by introducing Natural, Eco-Friendly habits into your daily routine.

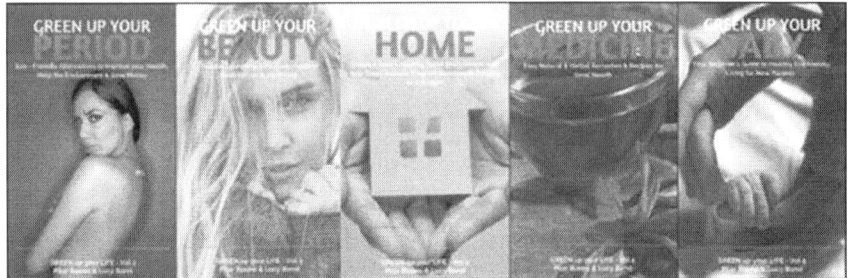

DOG TALES Series
Stories of Loyalty, Heroism & Devotion

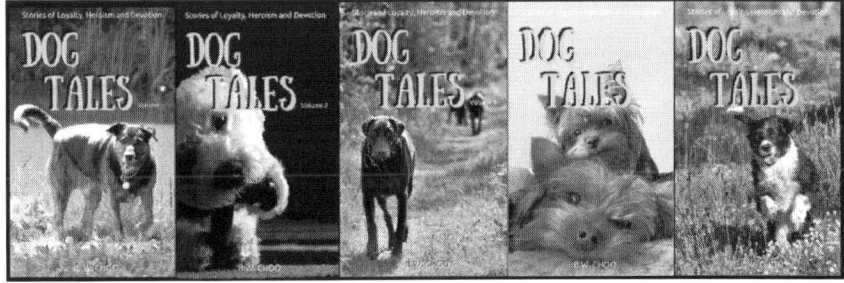

BUSINESS, INCOME & SOCIAL MEDIA Series
How to Promote, Market & Create Business with Social Media

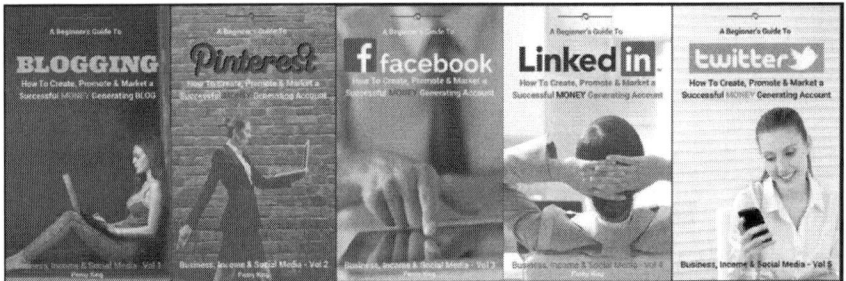

RESOLUTION TO BE HAPPY
Make yourself smile every day and banish stress and anxiety forever

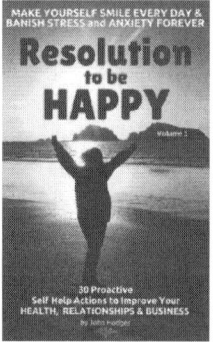

INTRODUCING GENETICALLY MODIFIED ORGANISMS - GMO
The History, Research and The TRUTH You're Not Being Told

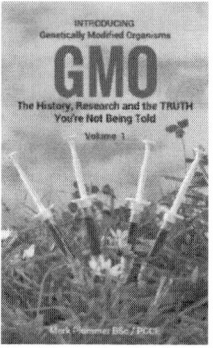

www.viddapublishing.com/books.html

Connect with John Hodges

If this book has helped you in any way or inspired you to take control of your own health and nutrition, it makes me a very happy man. For your Healthy, Nutritious, Green and Cruelty Free products, equipment and gadgets, don't forget to visit our online VIDDA Health Store: **astore.amazon.co.uk/vio7a-21**

If you have any questions at all, please feel free to contact me at: **viddapublishing.com/contact.html**

You can check out my publishing blog "Living like you mean it" (**viddapublishing.blogspot.co.uk**) for helpful tips, inspiration and updates on new books and free promotions coming soon:

You can also follow me on:

Twitter: twitter.com/VIDDAPublishing

John Hodges' Facebook: www.facebook.com/people/John-Hodges/550153788

VIDDA Publishing's Facebook: www.facebook.com/viddapublishing

Wishing you the best of Health.

John Hodges

John Hodge's Natural History Photography Archive:

www.pixelcashing.com/john-hodges

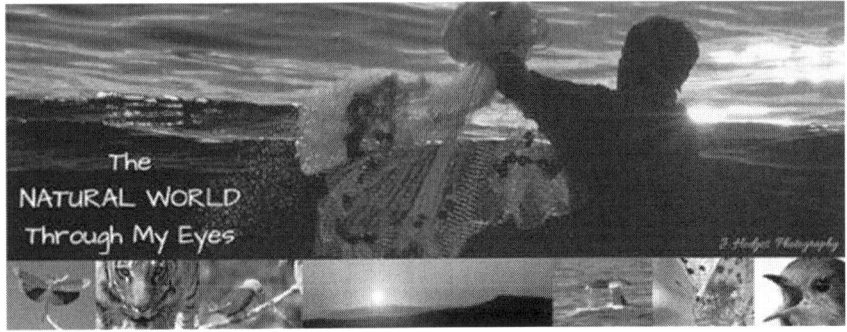

16688064R00053

Printed in Great Britain
by Amazon